THE YOUTH FORMULA

Outsmart Your Genes and Unlock the Secret to Longevity

Imagine a World Where Aging is Optional

NAVEEN JAIN

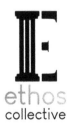

ethos
collective

Published by Igniting Souls
PO Box 43, Powell, OH 43065
IgnitingSouls.com

LCCN: 2024910115
Paperback ISBN: 978-1-63680-292-3
Hardcover ISBN: 978-1-63680-293-0
e-book ISBN: 978-1-63680-294-7

Available in paperback, hardcover, e-book, and audiobook.

Dedication

To those committed to living their healthiest life for as long as possible, may this book help you make smart decisions to put your health first, even when it's tough.

To my family, and colleagues and friends who are like family, I am deeply grateful for you.
Let's all stay young in body, mind, and spirit to enjoy many more years filled with joyful moments together.

And, to my Dad, thank you for giving me the courage to take on this journey while watching you battle cancer.

CONTENTS

FOREWORD

It won't be long now. By 2029–2035, people who are diligent about their health will reach the Longevity Escape Velocity, the moment in human history where we are adding more time to our remaining life expectancy than is going by. This phenomenon will be made possible by the exponential growth of technology and the convergence of Artificial Intelligence (AI) and biotechnology.

Forty years ago, I began tracking the growth of information technology and found the price-performance of computation was advancing exponentially. Whether measuring relay speeds, vacuum tube speeds, or integrated circuits, and regardless of whether the world was in war or economic depression, the exponential growth of information technology has remained steady. Since 1939, the price-performance of computation has increased over 75 quadrillion-fold, and it will continue.

This happens because information technologies make each next innovation easier, creating a feedback loop. For example, we use one chip to design a better chip.

Artificial Intelligence is now on track to reach human-level intelligence by 2029 and then quickly soar past us, a prediction I first made in 1999. As we begin to apply AI to every field, it is going to leap from transforming the digital world to transforming the physical world as well.

One of the most profound near-term transformations from AI is its impact on medicine. At the beginning of the COVID-19 pandemic, Moderna used a range of AI tools to help design and optimize mRNA sequences and discovered the sequence of their successful vaccine in just two days. They also used AI to speed up the manufacturing and testing process and saved countless lives. And very soon, AI will allow even more intensive biosimulations, rapidly testing billions of possible molecular sequences to find optimal medicines and reprogram our biology.

Nearly all functions of the body are carried out by proteins. They are the building blocks of life, and their unique individual shapes dictate the success or failure of all medicine. For fifty years, scientists tried to figure out how simple one-dimensional sequences of amino acids fold up into intricate three-dimensional proteins. This was called the Protein Folding Problem, and humans were unable to solve it.

Then, in 2022, AlphaFold 2, an Artificial Intelligence model created by Alphabet's DeepMind, shattered all expectations by predicting the structures of 200 million proteins, not just in humans but in all of nature. This marked a profound step forward in medicine because it unlocked information that scientists need to synthetically produce proteins with a desired function, for example, proteins that will stimulate our immune system to fight cancer.

The roadmap is clear: soon, we'll have the computational power to simulate organelles, cells, tissues, organs, and eventually the whole body. Instead of risky, expensive, slow clinical trials, we'll then be able to simulate trials digitally—a thousand times faster and tailored to each individual patient. The potential is breathtaking: to cure not just diseases like cancer and Alzheimer's but the harmful effects of aging itself.

Once we have Artificial General Intelligence at the end of the 2020s, medical advances will accelerate enough that people who are diligent with their nutrition, health habits, and using new therapies will reach Longevity Escape Velocity.

Right now, as you live through a year, you use up a year of your longevity. However, if you're diligent today about healthcare and nutrition, you might get back about three to four months per year from breakthroughs in scientific understanding. That is, you will only lose about eight or nine months of longevity in a year. However, AI progress is on an exponential curve and is speeding up every year. So, by 2029 to 2035, when you live through a year, you'll use up a year of your longevity, but you'll get back an entire year from scientific progress. And from that point forward, you will get back more than a year for every year you live so you'll be going backwards in time, as far as your health is concerned.

This is AI's most transformative promise: longer, healthier lives unbounded by the biological frailties that have limited humanity since its beginnings.

This book, by my friend Naveen Jain, provides a path to reach Longevity Escape Velocity at your peak health.

When he started Viome a decade ago, his mission was to make illness and aging optional. In these pages, he chronicles how he is getting there and how you can choose better health to extend your life. As you'll see, his solution is to delve into nutrition with the premise that if you eat the right foods and avoid the ones that impair your unique biology, you can avert gene expression that triggers aging and disease.

To get there, he has built a remarkable AI application that is focused on solving the big data problem. Viome now has the largest gene expression database in the world. Using AI, they can see patterns that have led to major health breakthroughs that were not possible before, even with a team of the brightest physicians, scientists, or researchers. Work of this nature is an essential step towards life extension, which I envision in three bridges.

In bridge one, we apply the moving frontier of current knowledge to slow down aging processes, emphasizing highly personalized approaches depending on your health situation. In bridge two, we will see the full blossoming of the biotechnology revolution when AI merges with medicine and unlocks the data we need to reverse and prevent aging. Innovators like Naveen are at the forefront of this revolution, leveraging AI to supercharge our health.

Finally, in the 2030s, we will reach bridge three, the nanotechnology revolution, in which medical robots—blood cell-sized computers—will augment our organs and immune system and ultimately connect our brains to the cloud. This is when we will break the shackles of our genetic legacy and achieve inconceivable heights of intelligence, material progress, and longevity.

Those who pursue optimal health today, using exponential technologies as they arrive, can expect extraordinary results. This includes Viome's AI engine, "Vie," which reliably predicts how specific foods will help or harm your microbiome, what nutrients you should eat for optimal health, and how to reverse any initial damage or early-stage health issues.

This book will teach you how to be diligent and provide a framework and formula for staying young as you age chronologically. It will help you take control of your own health so that you can see and experience the incredible future ahead, when the pace of technological change will be so rapid, its impact so deep, that human life will be changed forever.

—Ray Kurzweil

Health is the greatest of human blessings.

—*Hippocrates, Father of Western Medicine*

INTRODUCTION

Imagine it's your 100th birthday. You're at a party, and your closest family and friends are there. And although you've now hit the centenarian mark, you still feel like you're thirty. Your littlest great-great-grandchild toddles toward you with outstretched hands, and you scoop them up effortlessly and swing them into your arms. What a happy and extraordinary birthday!

Isn't that what most of us hope for? We want to be able to do what we want to do for as long as possible. That's the dream. But for most people the idea of picking up a 25 lb toddler at 100 is unfathomable. If we even make it to 100, wouldn't we be doddering and frail?

Certainly, when it comes to aging, there is a common trajectory that most people expect. Early signs of aging tend to appear around your 40th birthday. Vision goes. Energy declines. Stamina wanes. And you may encounter minor conditions that whisper to you: You're not young anymore. This comes with a hint of wrinkles, wisps of gray, and stubborn extra pounds. You start to believe that old age is coming, and you should prepare for decline. Then, by age fifty, if you're like most people, you will have one of four debilitating and ultimately fatal illnesses ahead of you—diabetes, heart disease, cancer, or a neurodegenerative disorder.

At middle age, we have been conditioned to look to the generation that came before us for clues about what the next two or three decades hold. What we see is visits to oncologists, cardiologists, and a bunch of other "ologists" and none of it is generally good news. But if you understand the emerging science today, you know that's BS. And if you don't, then it's a good thing you're reading this book.

This was the future that I was contending with in 2017 at the age of 57. I had just come out of my success with Moon Express, the first private company given permission to land on the Moon, so I was looking to take on a new audacious goal. And when I dug into the science of health and longevity, it became clear I needed to make it my mission. I started asking questions—the same ones you might be asking yourself since you're reading this book.

- Given today's technology, why can't we be healthy every day of our lives?
- Why are younger and more people getting sicker and dying from avoidable diseases despite the fact that interest in health and wellness is at an all-time high?
- How is it that human lifespans are still around 80 and not 180 or significantly longer?

So, I launched Viome, a company with a mission to make illness, and ultimately aging, optional.

Now, when it comes to tackling seemingly impossible problems, having no experience is a superpower. I was not an expert when I built Infospace, a web search company, in the early days of the Internet. Nor did I have any expertise in rocket science when I created Moon Express. When I started Viome, all I knew was that I wanted to solve a difficult problem that would benefit billions of people, including my colleagues, my family, and myself.

I quickly realized that my approach was fundamentally different from the current medical industry. I aimed to *solve* the problem of aging and disease, while today's medicine is primarily focused on managing symptoms rather than addressing their underlying causes. This system creates a dependency on temporary fixes, leaving people vulnerable. People have no tools for proactive lifelong health maintenance, and there is minimal support for health optimization and disease prevention.

It doesn't matter if you work in the system or use it as a patient; I'm sure you've experienced annoyances where you have questioned why healthcare is the way it is, especially when we have all this new technology and opportunity.

At the outset of my journey, I asked questions you might be asking as well:

- *Why do doctors still treat our bodies in separate parts?* The current system was built with a reductionist approach where the body is treated in components. How does this make sense, given that the body is a complex, unified system?

9

- *Why are there all these one-size-fits-all solutions when our bodies are all unique?* Generic solutions don't address individual needs, causing frustration, confusion, and potential harm.
- *Why are there more chronic diseases today?* Modern lifestyles do not support optimal health, including fewer nutrients in our foods. Why are more people not solving this?
- *Who can I trust when it comes to health information?* The commercialization of health and wellness prioritizes profit over genuine well-being. This creates confusion and mistrust, and people are not empowered to take control of their health.
- *Which technology tools should I use?* The rise of new health, diet, and fitness apps has overwhelmed people with data. This flood of often contradictory information lacks context, leaving people unsure how to interpret and use it.

While most of us hope that our doctors and institutionalized medicine will help us live longer, if we rely on them, we will die waiting. The system makes money when people are sick. It's not that people in the system are evil; it is just that no one is incentivized to keep us well. It's a massive problem that needs a fresh approach from outsiders. Innovation will come from entrepreneurs, not industry incumbents.

Approaching a topic as complex as longevity and health without any medical background has massive advantages. You have no preconceived notions about the sector you are stepping into, so you come to it with fresh eyes, clear thinking, and a healthy skepticism. You're also the one that asks the disruptive questions, which helps you uncover unconventional solutions and bypass institutional thinking. This counterintuitive approach produces breakthrough results.

I saw that we needed to approach the problem of human health in a different way. Why not tackle the challenges of health and longevity like a software problem and solve them using large biological datasets and artificial intelligence? Ultimately, the problem is a big data issue that we haven't had the tools to solve—that is, until now.

In this book, I am going to dispel many widely held beliefs that, thanks to recent science, are now considered invalid. Here are three:

1. **Your DNA is your destiny.** I will demonstrate this is not true. If your parents, grandparents, or siblings died too soon and younger than perhaps anyone hoped from a chronic condition, know that your genes are not a death sentence.
2. **Aging is not a choice.** I will show you that it is a choice. If you're experiencing signs of aging in your body, you can not only slow that process but reverse it.
3. **A disease-free life isn't possible.** I will show you how you can live your life disease free. If you're struggling with an illness or health issue, from acute to chronic, know that you can recover from it and live a fulsome and extended life. And you can continue to avoid any future disease states.

Has your skepticism kicked in yet? If it has, then I have a challenge for you.

As you read this book, and as I explain what we call *The Youth Formula™*, I ask you to put aside what you already know about health and longevity and give up your assumptions about your body, your medical history, your diet, your genetics, and what you think might happen to you as you age. Start from nothing. If I cover a topic you know something about, read it with an open mind. This is something I challenge myself to do daily, and it is one of the most important qualities in an entrepreneur who is setting out to rock the foundations of an industry.

I've discovered that when you do this, the impossible becomes possible, because you give up the constraints of what came before. You should also know that the ideas and approach here for a robust healthspan and a long life are not theoretical. The solutions are science-driven and backed by hard evidence.

This book is for anyone looking to stay healthy, optimize their healthspan, overcome chronic health issues, extend their lifespan, or address a health challenge. It also chronicles my journey building Viome as an entrepreneur, showing how to tackle complex, deeply ingrained problems with innovative thinking and a mission-focused approach. Entrepreneurs and emerging leaders will learn how to connect the dots in intricate systems, especially in healthcare, to create solutions that bring their dreams to life and make a significant impact on society.

But no matter what your "why," it is safe to say there is one reason we're all here. As Confucius once said: "A healthy man wants a thousand things. A sick man wants one."

The primary goal of this book is *awareness*. My aim is to empower and equip you with a new way to think about health, so you know what actions to take now and into the future to achieve an optimal healthspan, which means to *live a quality life for as long as possible.*

How to Read This Book

This book is designed to be read from beginning to end. You certainly can hop around chapters if you prefer. However, I have designed the flow of the book to explain my approach to health and longevity in an understandable and progressive manner. There is a significant amount of science and technology explained in these pages; however, I have done my best to make it understandable and interesting for the non-technical and non-medical reader.

For those who like to read quickly and digest the highlights, there is a summary of key points at the end of each chapter. And because I know people move fast these days, for the TL;DR crowd (Too Long; Didn't Read), I've called out the key takeaway from each chapter with a section I call "The Mindset Shift."

It is my wish that this book shifts your approach to your health in several ways, that it:

- Helps you to shift your mindset on health and aging by deepening your understanding of current science and available tools, which are critical for staying young.
- Teaches you how to ask better questions about your health, empowering you to take control and truly own it.
- Provides a practical Youth Formula to help you stay biologically young and healthy, even as you age chronologically.
- Simplifies the process of knowing what to do to stay healthy, making it easier to understand and achieve.

Oh, and one last thing: you may have noticed that the book's title, "Youth Formula," contains the word Y-O-U. This is intentional. There is no universal formula for youth that works for everyone. Instead, I'll show you how to use science and technology to decode *your* body so you can live a long and disease-free life. By understanding what your body uniquely needs and using the right tools to discover that, you can apply a you-centric approach—this is the true magic of the Youth Formula.

And then, that remarkable 100th birthday party can be your future.

—**Naveen Jain**

CHAPTER 1
WHAT IF AGING WAS OPTIONAL?

*The only way to discover the limits of the possible is
to go beyond them into the impossible.*

—*Arthur C. Clarke, Future, Inventor, Author*

My paternal great-grandmother lived until 106. From
what I remember of her, she was sharp and mobile until
the end. Her daughter, my paternal grandmother—my
Dadi—had a long life, too. She lived until 99.

When I left India in my early twenties, my family
followed, but Dadi stayed. Years later, I went to see
her as an adult. I vividly remember that trip. She was
in her final years and still active and engaged with the
family. She was walking and gardening every day. In
our conversations, she recounted every minor detail of
my stunts when I was a naughty and rebellious child. I

remember thinking how lucky I was to have her genetics. And you would think my father, her son, would have had a similar fate. But, as it turned out, that's not what happened.

At 82, my father died of pancreatic cancer. It's a type of cancer that's very difficult to detect. So, up to the day he got the diagnosis, we had no idea it was coming. He started complaining that his stomach hurt, and the doctor gave him antacids. By the time he had an MRI, as a precaution, we realized that he had cancer in his pancreas, and it was in Stage 4. He died not long after.

Before that, he had already survived prostate cancer. Then, a year later, he survived a heart aneurysm too. After these two incidents, his sub-functioning body continued to decline year by year.

Watching him die of cancer was heartbreaking. I will always remember him as a hardworking man who dedicated his life to his family, from which I have tremendously benefited. (Thank you, Papa.)

After my dad died, my mom, who is now 87, got more serious about her health. She has been hard at work using the approach in this book to address her various health issues, which include diabetes and high blood pressure. As for the rest of my family, my brother and sister have a high BMI, are obese, and take multiple pharmaceutical drugs. Yet, I am 65 and take no pharmaceutical drugs, have virtually no visceral fat, have high muscle mass, and my biological age is fourteen years younger than my chronological age.

Since I have the same genes as my siblings but a very different health profile, what gives? And how is it possible to have family members graced with a long and healthy life, yet have another that falls ill and dies too soon?

My motivation to crack the code on lifelong health stems from an innate obsession to solve big problems. I showed an early aptitude for this as a little boy. One day, my mother found me taking apart and reassembling a clock just so I could understand how it worked. My life has been full of puzzling through problems, though the "clocks" are getting more complex. My latest one happens to be longevity. And I plan to continue to solve problems like these until I am a very old man.

You may have come to this book for similar reasons: to be as healthy as possible for as long as possible. Or, perhaps you have not yet reached midlife but want to avoid declining health and maintain a resilient body as you get there. You may have also been diagnosed with a disease or condition you believe is possible to overcome.

It does not matter what category you fit into; there is one universal fact we can all agree on: there is nothing more humbling in this life than having a body that feels like it's working against you.

While we like to think our human intelligence makes us the smartest species on the planet—and some days we certainly think we're invincible!—once we develop one of the age-related diseases like diabetes, heart disease, or cancer, we quickly realize there's not much we can do. Life comes to a screeching halt when we grapple with our infirmity. Our bodies are the containers that allow us to do what we want. If they fail, we become limited in our abilities.

So, what if that never has to happen?

We already have evidence that avoiding illness and living long, healthy lives is possible. There are 90-year-old triathletes in this world and people who rarely get sick. We have superagers living to 100 and beyond. These people have a chronological age of 80, 90, or even 100, but their bodies on the inside are so healthy that their biological age is decades younger. Some people beat the odds, living longer and healthier lives than earlier generations. If some can do it, there must be a way we all can.

I want my grandmother's health and long life, and not the shortened health span that beset my father. I refuse it for myself and anyone else I can help. And my guess is, you want it too.

So, in 2017, I embarked on a mission to transform health and wellness. I launched Viome, a company dedicated to understanding the changes in our bodies that occur between being healthy and becoming ill. What causes us to age and succumb to disease? Viome aims to make illness and aging optional. Nearly a decade later, I am more convinced than ever that this vision is achievable.

Reimagining Health

In 2017, I came to a critical career-life juncture. I'd recently come out of a major success with my company, Moon Express, the first private company to get permission to go to the Moon. At the same time, I turned 57, which is when most people start thinking about retirement.

To me, the thought of retirement was terrifying. What would I possibly do? I suppose I could permanently move to my home in the British Virgin Islands to slow down and watch sunsets with my wife, a pastime I enjoy. But even as I put that in writing, it's a crazy thought. I have much to do in this life. I have a debt to repay. We all do. Especially if we have achieved great success, we must devote our time to a pursuit that moves humanity forward. Besides, I love to solve problems, so you can imagine how bored I would be sitting on a beach all day. Watching a fiery but fading sun descend a pinky-orange horizon is much better after a day of pursuing a goal that matters.

So, I asked myself what I could devote the next 10 to 15 years to. What mission could I possibly take on after achieving the massive goal of going to the Moon? The answer was surprisingly straightforward. I would take on the greatest problem facing humanity: The epidemic of aging and age-related chronic diseases.

Today, people are aging faster, getting sicker, and dying earlier from major avoidable chronic diseases. My father was one of them. Watching him die from cancer, a preventable illness, was especially hard because I couldn't save him, no matter how much I wanted to.

His story is not that unique. Instead, it's far too common. Aging today is a paradox. Rates of obesity, heart disease, and cancer are rising at a time when we've never had more abundance, possibilities, and opportunities. We have more affordable, accessible technologies and innovations than ever. How does this make sense? Here we are, living in the best of times, but we can't seem to stay healthy?

Obesity is a massive problem that continues to grow. Rates have tripled globally since the 1930s. More than 4 in 10 people are obese in the U.S. (the global rate is 38 percent).[1] As a precursor to many illnesses, it's likely the reason why, according to the statistics, noncommunicable diseases (NCDs) kill 41 million people each year. NCDs are chronic diseases like coronary heart disease, cancer, and diabetes. And they are completely *avoidable*. Yet, each year, 17 million people die from NCDs before age 70.[2] More than ever, we are likely to become obese, diabetic, or experience coronary heart disease or cancer. Or we'll succumb to a neurodegenerative disease like Alzheimer's or dementia or suffer major depression.

But these diseases don't happen overnight. We don't go to bed healthy and wake up with, say, Alzheimer's disease or bowel cancer. It may seem that way, but the onset of illness develops slowly over time. Our bodies send underlying signals long before symptoms appear. Minor issues like digestive problems and weight gain are often the first alerts of long-term chronic conditions. And while we've all heard (or used) the line, "It's in my genes," breakthroughs in science have taught us that's not the case. Lifestyle and nutrition is a far greater determinant of well-being. It comes down to what we eat and how we live each day. If we can understand our bodies more deeply and care for them, we can prevent aging and disease.

Our bodies send underlying signals long before symptoms appear.

I already had an inkling that lifestyle played a major role in longevity. My family had good genes: Great-grandmother, 106; grandfather, 100; grandmother, 99. My dad had their genetics, so what was different about his body that caused him to suffer two types of cancer and a heart aneurysm?

Early on, I realized one major difference was his Western lifestyle. Unlike his mother and grandmother, my father immigrated to America. He had access to a more modern lifestyle with greater technology and Western culture where processed foods were the norm and most packaged food products came with a large dose of sugar. Until he retired, he worked for the government as a civil engineer. Every day, he was always walking—about 10–15 miles a day at his work. But that stopped when he retired and moved to the United States, which is when his health began to decline. Unfortunately, it's a pattern I have witnessed in many others.

In retirement, many people lose their purpose. Then, there is a domino effect of decline. Everything starts to atrophy, including good habits. They no longer engage their brains, and they become significantly less active. Motivation flags. Once a person's purpose fades, they have less curiosity in life. They also find themselves around other aging people who also have this unfortunate mindset. Eventually, they look to the future, expecting more decline. Their body ages and does not process food as well. Nutrition is less of a focus. They start to feel isolated, suffer from pain, and deal with stress. Internally, what happens is cellular and molecular damage—which is what aging is—and this inevitably leads to chronic illnesses (in my Dad's case, pancreatic cancer).

As I dug into the problem, many people lamented to me that the healthcare system is broken. But it's not. The system is doing exactly what it was designed to do. The difference is that our *needs* have changed.

Our current healthcare system, created in the 1940s, was designed to keep people from dying from major infectious diseases.[3] And it does a great job of that. Once antibiotics were invented, many serious issues could be controlled. But now, new chronic diseases like diabetes, heart disease, and cancer are what take most people out. New times require new solutions. We have also learned that what were once great innovations like antibiotics, for example, have caused new health problems. In addition, our current healthcare system is designed to profit from unhealthy people. There is no money to be made if we're healthy. It's true no matter what country you're from. Most current-day healthcare systems are designed to treat you once you're sick or make you a subscriber for life by prescribing treatments for managing symptoms. There

> **Our current healthcare system is designed to profit from unhealthy people.**

are no system-wide strategies for optimal health and longevity.

But we also have never had as many advanced technologies and tools to understand our bodies. Artificial Intelligence and big data have already helped us do this. They are better at it than any human being. Today's capabilities to collect and synthesize biological data from millions of people, and eventually billions, is unprecedented. By contrast, we've historically had to rely on our doctors and their decades of experience with their patients. Think about it. The average family physician sees perhaps thousands of patients over a career versus millions of data points that can be processed by AI. Our insights into human health are staggeringly better today than they ever have been before. And in a decade or two? These last few decades are going to seem like the healthcare Stone Age.

Of course, we are not there yet. But there are already new solutions we can tap into. Since I've been on this journey, I have been using many to beat the odds. I am in my sixties and healthier than I was in my forties. I wake up at 5 am every day. I run up hills. I work an 80-hour week because I have the energy and the desire. Most people want to slow down and retire when they reach my age. But I am thinking about my next venture. I want everyone to live each day thinking about their future, as I do, and without consideration for how much time they have left.

I believe that in my lifetime, we will see that no one in the world needs to suffer from chronic diseases. This is the beginning of what we call precision health, a new, wild, and exciting frontier that presents a whole new set of questions that need to be answered. I am convinced that in the future, healthcare will be managed at home, not at a hospital. The medicines of the future will come from a farm and not pharmacies. Food can indeed be medicine, as Hippocrates said over 2400 years ago.

While we once had to treat our bodies as black boxes—simply counting calories or just eating the food we enjoy and hoping it would result in great health—now we don't have to. Thanks to converging new technologies, we have the ability to process, extract, and use highly personalized data to help us understand how our bodies work. Data makes the myriad of choices to improve our health clear. It's the core reason why, back in 2017, I launched Viome.

To date, we have built a software we call Vie, an AI engine that allows us to sort through mountains of data to help us understand what causes each individual to get sick and what nutrients the body needs to reverse it. Vie processes data sets beyond what the human brain (or all human brains working together) can comprehend. Using machine learning and other mathematical techniques, Vie is helping us make sense of the human healthscape and how to treat health issues when every person's body is biochemically different. And with every sample we process, Vie gets more sophisticated. Every day, we learn more and make important connections faster.

By the time this book goes to print, Vie will have analyzed over 1,000,000 samples. We will have amassed over 100 quadrillion data points (that's 100,000,000,000,000,000!). Viome currently has the largest gene expression database in the world. Already, it's led to many major health breakthroughs, allowing us to debunk many common health and nutrition myths.

A decade in, we are still in the nascent stage of learning about what causes aging and disease and how to mitigate both. Yet our work has yielded a flurry of insights that's allowed us to debunk common health myths and equip people with the insights they need to put their health back into their hands. I'll give you a snapshot of five common ones that will become more relevant for you over the course of this book as we dig into the science.

The Five Myths

Many individuals aren't leading their healthiest lives, largely due to prevailing socially accepted myths. My personal experience attests to this; before embarking on my health journey, I held several misconceptions about well-being truths. However, recent advancements in technology have ushered in new scientific insights. These developments have revealed that numerous health beliefs, widely accepted in the past, do not hold up under the scrutiny of modern science and data. As you'll see, when it comes to health, we have a great deal of unlearning to do.

Myth #1: Your DNA is Your Destiny

The blueprint in your cells—your "DNA"—does not predict health or longevity.

The makeup of your DNA shows the potential for everything that your genes are capable of and not what they are actually doing. Every cell in our body has the same DNA: our heart, our eyes, our nails, our neurons, our skin, our lungs, etc. Yet, we don't have eyes growing on our fingers and nails growing in our head. Why? It's because different parts of the DNA are over-expressed or under-expressed to make them different parts of the body. If DNA is like the alphabet, then what it expresses (RNA) is the story you write. Your lifestyle, the environment you live in, your stress levels, and what you eat can turn genes on or off.[4]

While most of us have been told that our genes are our destiny and that when we develop diseases, it's just "the bad cards we are dealt by the Universe," scientifically, that's not true. When we call it bad luck, we give ourselves a free pass. We avoid taking personal responsibility to enhance our health. Ultimately, great health is on us—our health destiny is fully under our control.

Less than 5 percent of diseases are genetic—they are called rare genetic diseases for a reason: they are rare. Genes play a very small role in most chronic diseases like diabetes, heart diseases, irritable bowel syndrome (IBS), inflammatory bowel disease (IBD), depression, or dementia.[5]

We now have the tools to identify threats in the body by analyzing our biological data. Using these results, we can gain insights into how to outsmart our genes so we can live healthier and longer.

Myth #2: There Are Universally Healthy Foods We Should All Eat

There is no such thing as a universally healthy food or diet. One-size-fits-all solutions don't work. Every person is unique and unlike any other person on the planet. The same food can have completely different responses, even in twins with identical DNA.[6] It's what your body does with food that makes it healthy or unhealthy for you. In other words, the adage "one man's food is another man's poison" has a literal meaning.

Take spinach, for example. It's often lauded as the ultimate superfood, and most people may not realize that it is also one of the leading dietary sources of oxalates—a group of compounds that, while naturally occurring, can bind to essential minerals and inhibit their absorption. In people whose gut microbiome can't digest oxalates, spinach can lead to kidney stones.[7] So, don't let anyone tell you that spinach is good for you—or grapefruit, or avocado, or broccoli, for that matter. I'll explain why in Chapter 4.

Now, before you clean those foods from your fridge in a panicked frenzy, know that they might be very good for you even though they may be bad for another person. Perhaps for you, they are superfoods.

Your body's response to food is as unique as your fingerprint.

Your body's response to food is as unique as your fingerprint. No two bodies are the same, so sweeping statements like "broccoli is good for you" are scientifically inaccurate. (Mom may have meant well, but our science shows she might have been wrong.) Same goes for almost all of the fad diets. If you're following a keto diet, paleo diet, or engaging in intermittent fasting, the truth is that you may be harming yourself.

Staying healthy is about knowing what your body needs at the molecular level and feeding it the right nutrients. In this book, you'll learn about the latest tools that can collect this type of information from basic biological samples (saliva, blood, and poop) that you can collect using at-home kits in about 20-30 minutes.

Myth #3: Slim People Are Always Healthy

There is a misconception that aesthetically pleasing and slim-looking bodies are synonymous with health. It's why the wellness culture is thriving. It's also why the weight loss industry generates almost $160 billion annually and is projected to grow to more than $305 billion by 2030.[8] Unfortunately, there are thousands of fast fixes for looking good that do damage over time. Our focus must be long-term health as much as we care about short-term results.

It's not about how much fat you have but what kind of fat you have. A person could be slim with high levels of visceral fat and liver fat (the most dangerous kind), and a person who is obese may have very little visceral fat but high subcutaneous fat (which is mostly cosmetic).[9] If you have followed fad weight-loss diets like keto, paleo, intermittent fasting, or any other diet that eliminates certain macronutrients, you may face serious digestive issues. These diets can completely disrupt your microbiome's ability to produce essential nutrients, leading to imbalances. Additionally, your hormone levels may become unbalanced, and your risk of heart disease and other chronic illnesses can increase significantly. Such diets have also been shown to accelerate biological aging.[10]

> A body that functions optimally on the *inside* leads to great energy, youthful skin, and a clear mind.

Just because a person looks thin doesn't mean they are well inside. A body that functions optimally on the *inside* leads to great energy, youthful skin, and a clear mind.

So, here's my counterintuitive approach you can borrow: when we make health a focus, beauty, energy, and youth are all byproducts we achieve.

Myth #4: A Declining Body Is an Inevitable Part of Aging, and There Is Nothing You Can Do About It

Most people believe that once we reach a certain age, we are certain to have declining health and low energy. There is a collective mindset—which has now been proven to be scientifically inaccurate—that we should expect our body to start to decline in our late thirties and into our forties and that it will progressively accelerate in the back half of our lives. Most people believe that decline and old age are *how it goes,* so you should accept that. Once you reach a certain age, you won't be able to do what you used to do. But that's not the case.

Have you ever asked yourself: *What is aging?* In a medical context, it simply means our body functions break down over time. This increases the risk of injury and disease, weakens our ability to fight infections, and eventually leads to death. This process speeds up when our body can't repair itself fast enough. Stress and poor nutrition make this worse by reducing resilience.

However, by managing stress and improving our body's repair and infection-fighting abilities, we can slow down aging significantly.[11] And now we have the technology tools to do that.

Living with most age-related diseases is a matter of choices you make every day, not bad luck. You don't need to suffer from illness or prolonged decline as you age. New technology can extend your healthspan, resulting in a longer, healthier life. Ultimately, staying young and vital is a matter of mindset and the lifestyle you choose. And part of that is knowing how to take

> Living with most age-related diseases is a matter of choices you make every day, not bad luck.

care of your body, given the science and technology of the day.

Myth #5: Illness or Aging is a Certainty

One of the most important dramatic lessons from a decade of puzzling through the mystery of human health and longevity might surprise you. There are about 40 trillion microbes in each of us. The activity of these tiny little symbiotic hitchhikers is a key determinant of whether we will get sick or experience aging decline. More than 99 percent of the genes in the human body don't come from a person's parents. They come from microbes that live in our gut, our mouth, and all over us.[12] Their interactivity with our body determines whether we live a truncated lifespan, like my father, or a long and healthy life, like my grandmother and great-grandmother.

These "bugs" (as they are sometimes colloquially referred to) are critical to living a healthy life. Collectively, they are known as your body's microbiome, and the medical community now recognizes it as an organ.[13] However, this newly recognized organ is under stress. Our modern lifestyle is causing microbial changes that are linked to increased risk of disease and accelerated aging.

Our industrial agriculture system uses harmful pesticides and synthetic fertilizers. We have many more foods and meats that are loaded with antibiotics to increase the shelf life of these foods (if we can even call it food). Our foods today are substantially less nutritious than they were a few decades ago.[14] Consequently, our bodies are getting less protein, calcium, and all the other vitamins we need to thrive. Our microbiome doesn't get what it needs to produce enough vitamins, minerals, and enzymes that our bodies need to stay healthy. For example, we need to eat eight oranges today to get the same benefits from eating one a decade ago.[15] Eight!

> **We need to eat eight oranges today to get the same benefits from eating one a decade ago.**

By thinking of our trillions of microbial allies as partners in our health journey, we can make more informed choices about our diet, lifestyle, and products we use. These microbes influence our resilience, immunity, and overall well-being. By nurturing a peaceful symbiotic relationship with them, we can harness their power to keep us healthy and potentially extend our lifespan. Embracing this holistic approach allows us to operate in harmony with our microbiome, optimizing our health and slowing the aging process. I believe the key to longevity may lie in how we care for and collaborate with these microscopic allies.

By changing the way we think and asking better questions about our health and why we get sick, we can create the new normal we need to be healthier. And ultimately, you'll come to understand what I now know: that while death may still be inevitable, lifelong health is a choice.

So, What is Possible?

The most beautiful words we've ever invented are "imagine" and "what if." When you say these words to another person, you have their attention, at least for a minute. They are words that let us suspend reality for the moment and contemplate a better one.

I always say that a problem worth solving is a problem that has an extensive impact on humanity and the future of our children. So, let's imagine if disease and aging were optional. What would be possible? What would it look like if people didn't get sick and spent their last decades in a working, viable body and not a broken and increasingly decrepit one? Can you imagine how our communities, our economies, and even our nations would flourish?

What if we redirected resources currently used to treat disease toward scientific pursuits that enhance our species' capabilities? The trillions of dollars we spend on health and wellness could be used to improve human existence. If humanity was free from the burden of disease, the cost of healthcare would be reduced on a global scale. Every country would save hundreds of millions, and even trillions, each year.

Of course, with extended lifespans, more people could live longer and use their wisdom to improve humanity. Imagine if retirement homes weren't designated for the old and sick but were places where legacy builders went to connect, flourish, and create in their final years.

What if most people lived until their last day with the same energy they had in their thirties? Imagine if diseases like heart disease, diabetes, or cancer were not the inevitable fate for the majority of people. What if anyone who became sick could easily get to the root cause, and they would know what lifestyle changes to make based on their body's data? A diagnosis would never be a death sentence; it instead would be a call to action.

Imagine that we knew how to maintain a healthy weight and look and feel young for life. Think of all the headspace we could free up! We could then pursue more important goals that improve the lives of others.

31

As each year goes by, I now believe this is increasingly possible. Aging will be optional. A disease-free life for anyone who wants one will be too.

How about you? What do you think is possible? Or what do you wish for? What do you want for yourself?

At the end of this book, I'll ask you again. In the meantime, keep these questions in mind as I take you through my journey and show you how my work and our team at Viome are making these promises possible. Bring along your doubts, your skepticism, and whatever concerns you have. By the time you get to the last page, I suspect you will realize that my counterintuitive approach might just be bang on.

The Mindset Shift

If you take one insight from this chapter, let it be this...

**You can have the body you want for as long as you want.
Optimal health and longevity is a *choice*.**

Key Insights

- When a person retires, their rate of decline will increase if they lose their sense of purpose in life. When a person doesn't have a "why" for living, it's easier to become complacent or to focus less on health.
- People are aging faster, getting sicker, and dying earlier from major avoidable chronic diseases. More than 4 in 10 people are obese in the U.S., and 74 percent will die from a major illness.
- Being a non-expert has an advantage for innovating in any industry. You can bring fresh eyes to a problem. You see what experts don't because they have been in a system for so long.
- There are no universally healthy foods. We need to eat what our bodies need, and those needs change over time.
- Your DNA is not your destiny. Lifestyle matters more than genetics, and this has been scientifically proven.

33

- A person with a thin body may not be healthy. What's happening inside is what matters.
- No one needs to accept decline as a natural part of aging. We now have affordable tools and more knowledge than ever to know what to do to stay healthy. Accepting aging decline is one way to ensure it happens because beliefs are self-fulfilling prophecies.
- If more people lived long, healthier lives, economies would thrive, and resources could be redirected to other areas of innovation. This future is possible.

CHAPTER 2
WHY THIS, WHY NOW, WHY ME?

Good health and good sense are two of life's greatest blessings.

—*Publilius Syrus, Philosopher, 43 BC*

In 2016, I was interviewed on television by a CNBC journalist about my company, Moon Express. Under the bright studio lights, I told the host (and the world) that my next company's sole purpose would be to make aging and illness optional. The problem is, I didn't set out to reveal that piece of news.

The interview focus was supposed to be on Moon Express's achievements. We were the first private company to receive permission from the U.S. government to land on the Moon, which attracted national media attention. The world wanted to know what we were doing, why we were doing it, and how an entrepreneur could do what only superpowers had done before. Before Moon Express, only governments could launch lunar missions. The U.S. and Russia had previously landed on the Moon under the Outer Space Treaty, a 50-year-old agreement between the two countries that governs space and forbids any nation from claiming sovereignty.

I answered all the expected questions about our mission to conduct mining on the Moon, and by the time the interview hit the four-minute mark, I figured we were nearing the end of my segment. Like most do, the host peppered me with questions to try and understand how I think. Going to space seems bold (or crazy, depending on who you ask). I told her there is no problem that entrepreneurship and innovation can't solve. And that led to the "what's next" question, a perennial media favorite. If you have been successful, everyone wants to know what's next for you. For me, of course, it was to figure out a way to slow aging and prevent disease.

Until then, I had only shared my next project around the dinner table and with a few close business friends. My inner circle said it was smart but crazy, which, to me, was great news. They are the people who know me best, so when they think I'm insane, they also know I have a track record for success and that I plan to make it happen.

To my surprise, the CNBC interview wasn't over. Hearing my plan, the host pressed me about how I planned to slow aging and prevent disease. Her first response was a "Wow…" and then it was followed by a stream of questions: "How do you suppose that's possible?" "What do you plan to do?" "Have you started?" I'll never know for sure what she was thinking, but based on her expression, it was something like: *The dude is crazy. But wait, he may be onto something. He did build a company that became the first private company to leave Earth's orbit and go to the Moon.* So, for a minute more, I shared my idea and plan (which wasn't much yet). I told them I would solve this audacious challenge and that we have to think differently and ask a new set of questions.

Critics said landing on the Moon was nothing compared to what it will take to eliminate chronic disease. Still, extraordinary things happen when you make a public declaration, as I did that day. When you choose an audacious moonshot, the Universe conspires to help you. Once you commit and begin to share your vision, top experts are drawn to your mission. They gravitate toward you because they seek purpose and a lasting legacy, not just money. They want to work on solving the world's biggest problems. The very idea you're pursuing becomes a source of inspiration, attracting the right people to your project. And that is exactly what happened next.

But before we delve into what followed, let me first share my thought process on selecting the audacious project to which I have dedicated the next two decades of my life. This will be of special interest to readers who are entrepreneurs or business leaders.

Any time you attempt to innovate, evaluating your idea is a crucial first step. It helps you understand the resources required, the expertise needed, and the connections you'll want to forge. In the complex realm of healthcare, this has meant grasping the intricacies of the current system and collaborating with pioneering scientists on the front lines of research. This careful evaluation is what I do in all businesses. It sets the foundation for attracting the right people and aligning the necessary elements to achieve your bold vision.

You will learn the process I go through when I approach solving a new problem and how you, too, can think differently, not only about your health, but also your own life's mission. By challenging the foundations of what has come before, we can unlock new pathways to a healthier, more fulfilling future.

With any major problem, there is always someone who has to stand up and say, "Hey, there is a better way to do this." That is leadership. We can't just wait for change. We need to act and use the tools available today to tackle chronic disease and aging. It always takes someone to be the "crazy" catalyst.

Beyond the Moon

> When I think about problems in our world, I think of what *can be*, not what is.

When I think about problems in our world, I think of what *can be*, not what is. Most people get caught up in the here and now, focusing only on what's directly in front of them. Their perspective narrows, and their vision becomes short-sighted. They react out of fear, and over time, they adopt a mindset of limitations, forgetting to see the world with the boundless curiosity and possibility they had as children. They lose sight of their dreams and what is truly possible.

Over the years, I've learned that when you start practicing the art of visualization, your mindset shifts from "This is impossible" to "What do I need to achieve this?"

This transformation opens up a world of possibilities and fuels the drive to turn dreams into reality.

Seeing beyond what exists today and pushing the boundaries starts with asking the right questions. So, every time I start a company or devote my time to a major pursuit in my personal life, I ask myself three questions. It's a process I call Know Your Whys.

I always ask:

1. Why this?
2. Why now?
3. Why me?

These questions were how I explored the problems and mechanics of why we age and get sick. It's where it became evident that innovations were possible.

Let's start with "Why this?"

Why This?

I always start by asking, "Why this?" Then, I fast forward in time and imagine the problem I set out to solve is now resolved. Next, I ask, "Would solving this problem help a billion people live a better life?" If the answer is yes, that's a signal I'm on the right track. This process helps me determine if the problem is worth my time, commitment, and energy.

Helping a billion people is about doing good in the world but also about purpose and personal fulfillment. There is no greater motivating force than a problem that helps a billion people. When you have a goal like that, you want to get out of bed every day. You go to sleep knowing that what you're doing matters. Every day, you feel you are living a life well lived. It doesn't matter what happens in your day, good or bad; you've won.

Most importantly, I know that if you build a product or service that helps one billion people live better lives, you have automatically created a hundred billion-dollar company. And with that success, you can help even more people by creating an even bigger company. Your focus needs to be on helping more and more people rather than on making more money. You see, making money is a byproduct of improving lives.

So, when you wake up in the morning, ask yourself: What can I do today to improve other people's lives? Then, you have a kernel for creating a large, successful enterprise. Even if you're not building a business, you can still use this principle to orient yourself to join the right mission.

So, "Why this?" was the first question I asked when I considered diving into the healthcare industry.

As I mentioned earlier, I'd just succeeded with my company, Moon Express. It was the first private company to receive permission to leave Earth's orbit and land on the moon. Moon Express was a massive goal achieved, and it is what I call a moonshot.

Moonshots are ideas that most people think are difficult at best and, at worst, impossible to achieve. They are worthy causes and the only goals anyone should want to spend their time on. When humans challenge the boundaries of what we believe is possible and succeed, we push humanity forward. You can learn more about this approach in my first book, *Moonshots*. But for context, we'll define it again here because it also applies to our mission to take on aging and illness.

Moonshots are massive and seemingly impossible missions like human flight. In the late 1800s, many scientists claimed humans weren't meant to fly. They said planes could never take off; it was considered impossible. Before that, people thought cars would never go faster than horses because some believed the human body would explode or, at minimum, suffer significant harm.[15] It's ridiculous to imagine this was once the accepted truth, yet it is understandable given the times. People had never seen anything faster than a horse. So how could they believe the human body could travel 50 miles per hour, in the case of an early car, or 400 miles an hour in an aircraft? They certainly thought pilots would perish. Yet, both of these barriers were shattered, and into the 21st Century, we continue to find ways to propel ourselves ever faster. The current land speed record is 763.035 mph, achieved in 1997.[16] The record for fastest traveled goes to the crew aboard Apollo 10, which, in May 1969, achieved a speed of 24,816.1 mph.[17] And no bodies exploded.

Another classic example is Roger Bannister, the first middle-distance athlete to run the first sub-four-minute mile. He showed the world that it could be done in three minutes and 59.4 seconds when it was thought impossible. At the time, the idea was that the human body would fall apart if it ran any faster. But Bannister did it, and eleven people achieved that speed the next year after he did it.[18] Suddenly, people could do something that had yet to seem achievable. How? Because they believed it was possible.

The human mind is so powerful that it creates limitations it believes are insurmountable. In other words, we limit ourselves if we're unwilling to question our thinking. The best approach to life is to embrace an abundance mindset. And you'll find that thinking this way gets you closer to thinking in line with reality, including great health. If we don't believe it's possible to have the body we want and be healthy until the end of our lives, our behavior will reflect our disbelief.

When I ended my time at Moon Express, I asked myself: What do you do for an encore after you complete a literal moonshot of going to the Moon? As I searched for an answer, it became obvious. Start another moonshot! But this time, it had to be symbolic.

A symbolic moonshot is a problem that humanity has yet to solve because it seems impossible. Or, more accurately, because no one is asking the right questions. Examples of symbolic moonshots today are companies like OpenAI, which has a mission to ensure that AI benefits humanity. It's certainly done with innovations like ChatGPT, its famous AI language model trained on large internet datasets. It helps the world access instant answers, write computer code, or write better and faster.

Google is another company that has a symbolic moonshot. It organizes all the information on the Web to make knowledge universally accessible. It's become so woven into our lives that it's a verb. How many times have you had a problem and "googled" it? Another positive industry disruptor that comes to mind is Mindvalley, a transformational education company that is raising human consciousness. We've collaborated on online courses to encourage more people to embrace entrepreneurship and improve their health and lives.

When I considered my symbolic moonshot, I considered our biggest problem today and realized that there is no greater problem than the epidemic of aging and disease.

Last year, the U.S. spent $4.7 trillion on healthcare[19] and $4.4 trillion on wellness products and services.[20] Yet, our rates of obesity, disease, and early mortality are the highest for a country like ours. We have the highest maternal and infant mortality among Western nations. We also have the highest death rates for avoidable or treatable conditions like cancer, diabetes, heart disease, and neurological disorders.[21] These are also known as the Four Horseman diseases and are the reason most people die earlier than they have to. We also know that these chronic illnesses are completely avoidable.

We can no longer blame our genetics. Even if your mom or dad died from one of these diseases, it doesn't mean you have to. Yet, today, we have more people with multiple chronic conditions than ever. We also have more people struggling with obesity, which is a key risk factor for chronic conditions such as diabetes, hypertension, other cardiovascular diseases, and cancer.

Every year, the U.S. spends approximately 17.8 percent of its gross domestic product (GDP) on healthcare. That is nearly twice the amount of other Organization for Economic Co-operation and Development (OECD) nations, which are countries that contribute to key global issues. As a share of GDP, our healthcare expenses per person continue to be far higher than other high-income countries. And by 2031, our total spending is projected to rise to $7.2 trillion. Our wellness spending is also growing. By 2025, it's projected to grow to $7 trillion.[22] Specifically, it's been suggested that Americans spend about $60 billion each year on diets trying to lose weight. At the same time, 90 percent say they don't get results.[23] So, then, who is benefiting from the growth of the health and wellness economies?

I did the research on other countries, too; for those readers who live in a country outside the U.S., I learned that while some measure higher on global reports, there is still nowhere in the world where the basis for health and wellness is focused on optimization and longevity. No nation's current healthcare system proactively prevents illness before it arises, optimizes lifelong health, or focuses on eradicating sickness entirely. Foundationally, the design of the system is flawed. Even in countries that top the list of best healthcare globally, such as Saudi Arabia, Japan, and the United Kingdom,[24] the ethos that underpins every system is sick care. It's even in the label. Healthcare is about "care," not optimization.

Since its inception, healthcare, particularly in the West, has been a "wait and see" game. The nature of the system is reactivity, not proactivity. We get treatments when symptoms show up. If we're not in trouble, we're fine with only a yearly checkup to ensure everything is in tip-top shape. When we do receive treatment, it's to make symptoms disappear. Other times, all that can be done is symptom management. Our current system helps us maintain average. Because, generally, getting to the root is not cheap.

Achieving optimal health and avoiding aging and disease requires more effort. Illness starts long before symptoms. No one eats a tub of fried chicken, clutches their heart, and keels over on the spot. Deterioration of the heart starts years before an attack. Similarly, no one goes to bed and wakes up dying of thirst because suddenly they have type 2 diabetes. It's a road that involves years of unhealthy habits. The same is true of neurodegenerative disorders. Brain signals and regions deteriorate over time. We need a way to detect decline long before it happens. And given the technologies available to do so, there is no doubt it's possible.

At this point, we need to take a deep breath and ask: How can people be getting sicker, aging faster, and dying younger from avoidable diseases at a time when we have more advanced technological tools? We live in a time when there has never been so much access and innovation. When I thought about this back in 2017, it was clear we needed a new solution.

Most of us want to live our healthiest lives for as long as possible. For me and my Viome colleagues, our mission has never been about living forever. It was about being healthy as long as we live. Who wants to live a long time if you're sick? Early on we realized longevity also needs redefining. Who wants to live long if you don't feel good? So the question we were trying to answer was: why can't we stay healthy until the day we die? It doesn't matter how old we live; it could be 100 or 150 years with our technological advances. Why can't we be healthy until the very end?

Why can't we stay healthy until the day we die?

As we age, chronic diseases tend to become part of our life. We become obese or diabetic, or we suffer coronary heart disease, cancer, or one of the neurodegenerative diseases. But as I started to learn, all of these illnesses have a theme: chronic inflammation, which causes chronic disease. I wondered: *What if we could understand what changes in the human body occur when you develop chronic diseases? What changes as we age? And what if we can use nutrition and other lifestyle choices to prevent and reverse aging and illness?*

At that point, I'd answered, "Why this?" Nothing was more important than focusing on health, which touches us all and is a matter of life or death.

But was it the right time?

Why Now?

I always ask, "Why now?" because it helps me focus on timing to see if a market is ready for innovation. Could we build an affordable solution that allows us to live healthier and longer and avoid aging and disease?

Asking "Why now?" is about considering what has changed in the last two to three years and what will likely happen in the next three to five years to solve a problem at scale. Whatever you take on shouldn't be a problem that could have been solved five years ago. If the tools to solve it are available, but the problem has yet to be solved, it's likely because there is no need for the solution or the technology required has yet to catch up. In short, you want to intercept tomorrow's emerging technologies now to solve tomorrow's problem. Using yesterday's technologies to solve tomorrow's problems is a futile pursuit.

Over the years, I've learned that the number one predictor of business success differs from what most people think. Many entrepreneurs emphasize having a great idea. Or they believe the key is to find the best solution to a problem. I've also seen entrepreneurs claim that focusing on using the best technology to solve the problem is key. Others say winning in business is a result of a high-performing team. Those are all valid to varying degrees. But the number one predictor of success is timing. One study tracked over 150 companies and over 45 IPOs and acquisitions and found that timing accounted for 42 percent of a business's success.[25]

Examples of this are companies in the sharing economy, like Airbnb and Uber. Airbnb is well-known for disrupting the hotel industry. It is a winning idea now, but that was not the case at one time. When it was first pitched to investors, a person renting their home to a stranger seemed ludicrous. Many early VCs passed on Airbnb. They did not think vacationers would want to stay in a person's home or that homeowners would want to rent space to a stranger. Airbnb also had a very good business model. Still, that did not lead to its success. The win for Airbnb was timing. The company launched during a recession. People needed money to such an extent that they dismissed the perceived concerns and inconveniences of renting their homes.[26]

Uber is another well-known disruptor that succeeded due to timing. While it also had a great business model and strategy, it was a radically new idea. Having ordinary people transform their cars into taxis seemed a bit odd. Uber succeeded because it came at the right time. Drivers wanted to make extra money, so taxiing people in a private vehicle and taking bookings via mobile phone seemed appealing. It was a simple solution for people to make more cash.[27]

So, as I considered "Why now," I paid close attention to trends in the health and wellness industry and conducted extensive research. It was then that a clear pattern emerged: the microbiome was connected to nearly every disease and was featured in hundreds of research papers.

Recognizing its significance, I sought technology capable of analyzing both microbial and human gene expression while also exploring other technologies that could expedite finding the answers I needed.

I also noticed the cost of genome sequencing was coming down. In 2017, it cost approximately $1,450. Only seven years prior, it was $50,000, and most people could not afford to get their genome sequenced. But seven years later, it was within reach of most middle to upper-middle-class consumers. Over the years, I've watched the price drop as technology became more sophisticated and more companies entered the space. I figured it would finally reach $100 in two or three years, which is where we are today. As of writing this book in 2024, some companies sequence the genome for as little as $100 to $200.[28] Now, these are retail prices, so the base cost to sequence a genome is really tens of dollars.

When we started Viome, I thought our projection was ten times more optimistic than what actually happened. As it turns out, given the current wholesale cost has reached $10 per sequencing, we were ten times pessimistic!

To me there was now this perfect storm for innovation. I had this problem of understanding aging disease where the link appeared to be related to the microbiomes. And sequencing costs were coming down so we'd be able to do something that was affordable for the masses. In addition, to make sense of the data, the processing power became sufficient because AI capabilities had improved.

As an innovator, I have learned it's important to remember how technological growth fools most people and avoid being fooled yourself. While people think linearly, technological growth is exponential. Each iteration uses what's previously been created to build the next. This is why technology accelerates faster over time and why the time between innovations gets shorter.

Computers are a great example. Early computers were room-sized in the 1950s and 1960s and became cabinet-sized in the 1970s.[29] A decade later, companies came out with computers that could fit on a desk. This innovation sparked the personal computer revolution. With computers becoming more accessible, more people had access to them. They became powerful tools that could complete many day-to-day tasks faster than ever before, connecting people and bringing information to the masses.

In the 1960s, Gordon Moore, one of the co-founders of Intel Corp., noticed that the number of transistors in computer chips was doubling every one to two years.[30] A transistor is a tiny switch made of silicon that is used by computer chips to interpret and process data. Simply put, it's how ones and zeros are translated into images and text on a screen. Computers have become faster because, over time, humans have been able to make smaller transistors and fit more of them on every computer chip. This doubling makes computers faster.

A few years ago, we weren't sure this doubling would continue due to the physical limitations of miniaturization. You can't shrink transistors smaller than the molecules they are made of. Technologists thought at some point we wouldn't be able to make these switches any smaller, but we did. Then, quantum computing emerged. It harnesses the unique properties of quantum physics to process information in a fundamentally different way than traditional silicon processors. Unlike classical computers, which use bits that are either 0 or 1, quantum computers use quantum bits, or qubits, which can exist in multiple states simultaneously.

So, the technology innovation gap between iterations of devices continues to shrink. What used to take 1000 years to improve decreased to 500, then to a century or so, and then it shrunk to decades. In the second half of the 20th century, transistor-powered processors (and later Intel's microprocessors), shortened the innovation time scale to months. Today, the space between improvements in most technologies has been reduced to less than a year. In some cases, the time span is seasonal. It's why the smartphone you bought in the spring is a generation behind once autumn arrives.

People have a tough time comprehending exponential growth. It's because our brains think linearly.[31] We process information in a straightforward, orderly, and sequential way. We think similarly to how we climb stairs. Most of us start at the bottom and walk up the flight step-by-step at a consistent pace until we reach the top. Exponential steps would be more like riding an elevator. You get on, and the elevator moves you initially at a slow speed but accelerates until you are zipping faster toward the next floor.

Meanwhile, the human brain is wired for survival. It developed to handle close-by, straightforward, and mostly unchanging situations. It's how we stayed safe when we were cave people roaming the Earth without cars, mobile phones, or GPS to get us from here to there. We've evolved to think linearly. Unsurprisingly, our organizations, social systems, and government institutions are designed using this same thinking model. We have hierarchies, escalating grade scales, and capital systems.

When I explain the difference between linear and exponential growth, I often use two simple examples: one with steps and the other with money.

Imagine we're standing together in a room, and I ask you to take thirty linear steps. How far would you go? Think about it now. If you're like most people, you'd probably say you'd be by the door or halfway to it. You would take step 1 and then 2 and walk in sequence. But what if it was thirty exponential steps? At this point, most people do some quick math. They add up the steps, but now they double them—2, 4, 8, 16. They figure maybe they'd get outside the building or downtown. But thirty exponential steps would take you 16 times around the Earth! Here is the difference using only 10 of those thirty steps:

Ten linear pairs of steps:
2+4+6+8+10+12+14+16+18+20 = 110 steps
Ten exponential pairs of steps:
2+4+8+16+32+64+128+256+512+1024 = 2046 steps

It is hard to fathom a number as large as thirty exponential steps. The same happens when we compare money. Would you rather have $100 million in your bank account or start with $1 but double the amount in the account each day? Do some quick math, and you might initially think you'd never get to a million using the $1 doubling option. But 31 doublings later, the account would hold more than $1 billion.

Day 1 = $1
Day 2 = $2
Day 3 = $4
Day 4 = $8
Day 5 = $16

After Day 7, you'd have $64. After Day 15, you'd have $16,384. By Day 30, you'd find $536,870,912 in your bank account. And on the 31st day, you'd have more than $1 billion on deposit.

The bottom line is technology grows deceptively fast. So, many people see rapid growth but generally don't get concerned. The growth feels sequential. But then, the growth trajectory hits the knee of the curve. It takes off. People look at each other and say, where did that come from?

Linear versus exponential growth looks like the graph in Figure 2.1.

Figure 2.1: Linear versus exponential growth

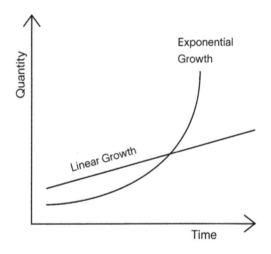

People think in a linear fashion while technology grows exponentially, accelerating over time.

We saw this progression with technologies like 3D printing. It slowly puttered along, and then boom. Today, it's one technology that has and will continue to change the world. Or think of voice recognition that was once speaker-dependent. A system that understood a Texan wouldn't work well for a speaker from Chicago. Today, you can speak to a personal assistant like one of the devices in most languages in any accent, and the device will understand you and provide an answer back in a few seconds.

It's why many feel the level of change we're experiencing today is perplexing and increasingly disorienting. But this is good news. It means we can get better results much faster over time. It's also why almost every facet of society is being disrupted and reinvented. Understanding exponential technological growth helped me see that healthcare would be one important area in need of reinvention.

Today, in medicine, there is a tremendous focus on treating symptoms, not root causes. Many companies, too, are focused on symptom treatment rather than eradicating disease. As I dug deeper into healthcare, I learned that our medical industrial complex makes money when we are sick and makes no money when we are healthy. Think about it for a second. Our healthcare system has no incentive to keep us healthy. It's not that people want to hurt others, but rather, the way the system is designed is that people are incentivized to make money off the wrong thing.

If you have an autoimmune disease, for example, you're likely to be prescribed a drug that will suppress the immune system instead of getting to the root of why your immune system is attacking you. (This happened to our Chief Science Officer, Momo, by the way.) These drugs make it easier for a patient to get an infection. If it doesn't work for you, the solution in the current system is to prescribe a different drug.

Today, more people are waking up to this truth and looking for answers outside of the traditional doctor's office that's about waiting until you get sick. People are also more focused on longevity and staying healthy both physically and mentally. With the growth and access to more technological tools and customization in other areas—our homes, when surfing the internet, and when purchasing online, people want personalization. Personalization is going to be expected at some point, not just a luxury, and we have the technology to make this possible in everything.

Imagine what would be possible if people were empowered and had the tools to know what to do to stay healthy. What if 80 percent (or more) of the population stayed healthy until they died? They'd monitor themselves regularly and perhaps get an annual physical to stay well. Now, let's say only a small fraction of those people have a chronic illness that requires medicine. A healthier population would result in fewer doctors, hospitals, and pharmaceutical companies. Think of all the people who could refocus their time, effort, and resources on solving others' problems to benefit society.

At this point, I realized it was on me or someone like me to get involved. When considering "why now?" my answers pointed to the sweet spot I always need to launch a company. To this, I will leave you with an adage from hockey (coined by Wayne Gretzky's father, Walter) that's often used in business: Skate to where the puck will be, not where it has been. I realized it was time to lace up.

The last question, then, was, "Why me?"

Why Me?

I always ask, "Why me?" because this part of my process is about considering I am approaching the problem differently than anyone else.

If you use this same process, it's important to make sure that you are asking questions that no one in the industry is asking. Remember that the questions you ask are the problems you solve. Changing the question allows you to look at the problem differently and opens up the possibility of solutions that weren't obvious before.

For instance, people often talk about solving world hunger. They think it's about growing more food, improving the distribution of food to get it to more people, or minimizing food waste during transportation. But what if we asked a different question? What if we ask: Why do we eat food? You suddenly realize that we need food as a source of energy to fuel our body and to provide nutrition. What are the different ways we can get energy?

Plants get energy from photosynthesis and there are bacteria that thrive in radio-active nuclear waste. That means these bacteria have figured out how to protect themselves from the intense radiation but also are able to use radiation as a source of energy. What if we can take genetic material from these bacteria and use CRISPR to modify our genes so we are both protected from radiation and are able to use radiation as a source of energy? Imagine asking your partner about going out for radiation and not for pizza! *Honey, would you like to go to Radiation Hut?*

As I dug into the illness and aging dilemma, I started to see it in a very different light. I had an edge because I was an outsider to the industry. I was like a kid incessantly asking, "Why?"

At the time, scientific communities were focused on DNA. There was this idea that if you knew your DNA, you would know how your body works, and you would be able to find out how long you would live and how to stay healthy. So, everyone wanted to do DNA testing. In 2018, DNA tests by companies like 23andMe and Ancestry were all the rage. They were so popular that 26 million people had purchased a consumer DNA test by the end of that year.[32] The trend was partly because of emerging science but also due to a heavy media focus on the trend.

You might remember when Oprah featured a segment on DNA tests on her show *Super Soul Sunday*. There was a short segment at the end of an episode where strangers from different countries gathered to do their DNA tests. The group learned they were more closely connected than they thought. It featured a staunch Brit who dislikes Germans and later discovers he is part German. There was a woman who said she didn't love Turkish people and turned out to be of Turkish descent. Two people in the group learned that they were cousins. Eyes bulged out of their sockets, and there were hugs and tears. Viewers watching from home learned we are more alike than different.[33]

These DNA tests, which cost as little as $59, can give clues to who your third cousin is and perhaps some insight into why you like savory over sweet or if you have the potential to develop a rare genetic disease. But I realized DNA cannot tell you if you are healthier now than you were a year ago. DNA also won't provide insights into how your body functions or identify which foods might spike your glucose levels, potentially leading to diabetes.

As I dug into DNA science as a non-medical expert, I started to ask new questions that needed to be asked. I realized that your genes don't change when you develop most chronic diseases. Let's say you gain 200 lbs and get diabetes. Your genes (DNA) will still be the same. Or perhaps you develop heart disease. Again, your genes have stayed the same. DNA is the same from birth to death for every human. A baby's DNA is the same at birth as it is as they grow into an adult, and it is still the same at the end of the person's life.

This was the "ah-ha!" moment for me. If DNA can't tell you if you are dead or alive, how will it tell you if you're becoming healthier or sicker? There had to be another answer. I soon learned there was.

Your genes (DNA) don't change, but your *gene expression* (RNA) is constantly changing as we develop obesity, diabetes, depression, heart diseases or cancer.[34] What genes are overexpressed or underexpressed or even turned on or turned off determines your health and longevity. And if we can identify what factors were impacting expressions of our genes, we could get ahead of it and can help people avoid these triggers to live healthier longer.

> Your genes (DNA) don't change, but your gene expression (RNA) is constantly changing as we develop obesity, diabetes, depression, heart diseases or cancer.

Asking the right questions led me to understand the critical role of RNA in health, how to measure health over time, and how to develop active, personalized health solutions. These insights were foundational to Viome. Coupled with the perfect timing and the advanced technologies available to scale our health solutions globally, our path forward became unmistakably clear.

Your Genes Aren't Your Destiny

A myth that has been firehosed into most of us is the belief that our genetics are our destiny. We now know that is not true.

It's so ingrained that, for many, it's the default answer to any health issue. We tend to go to our family tree when we get a symptom. "If my parents have heart disease (or diabetes, or depression, etc.), then I am destined to develop that chronic disease when I get to their age," you might say, or "If obesity runs in my family, I'm stuck with this body." We often buy into ideas, believing that the fate of our grandparents and parents is likely to be ours, and then it becomes a self-fulfilling prophecy. We give up because of our genes, not realizing that a person's lifestyle is more important than their DNA and that we can control our gene expression (RNA) based on the foods we eat and our lifestyle choices. Most people do not realize that the daily decisions we make affect our gene expression, and this is what leads to dis-ease of the body.

So, why do most people think they're genetically pre-destined to get some familial condition? It was simply what was once believed. A grandparent died of a particular disorder, then we saw a parent develop the same illness, and we figured we were next. Then, at the turn of the 21st century, scientists discovered that our genes are not our destiny.

You might remember in the late nineties and early 2000s, scientists initiated the Human Genome Project (HGP). It was an ambitious research effort designed to decipher the chemical makeup of the entire human genetic code and gain an understanding of human DNA. In April 2003, the research team generated the first sequence of the human genome.[35] It was one of the most remarkable scientific achievements in history, a milestone that provided crucial insights into the blueprint of humanity. The work significantly advanced the study of human biology and the practice of medicine.

Scientists learned that the human body has approximately 23,000 protein-coding genes.[36] In simpler terms, this means we have 23,000 bio-blueprints that are coded with instructions for making the proteins essential for many functions of our body. The body uses proteins as building blocks to grow muscles, fight diseases, and manage our metabolism. It was a major breakthrough that led to a startling revelation.

The finding that humans have 23,000 genes initially confused scientists. That number is surprisingly small, especially considering how complex human beings are. For example, the genomes of house plants have similar gene counts. A rice plant has 46,000 genes, double that of humans.[37] We have fewer genes than the remnants of a half-eaten sushi roll. How does that work? And how are we so sophisticated? The answer came from understanding the tiny organisms that live within us.

If we look at the genes of the approximately 40 trillion microbes in and on our bodies, we see that theirs outnumber ours by about 100 to 1. Each microbe encodes 3,000-4,000 genes.[38] Once we include our microbes in the total gene count, it makes sense that we are more sophisticated than a basic food staple. This also means that 99 percent of all the genetic material in our body doesn't come from our mom and dad.[39] At best, we are 1 percent human, which begs the question: who controls whom? Could we primarily be a portable ecosystem for a microbial society? It's mind-boggling. The bacterial genes that are referred to as the human microbiome have such an influence on physiological regulation that the medical community recognizes them as an additional organ.

People have this idea that they might have a gene that causes Alzheimer's and will suddenly wake up one day when they are 50 or 60 years old to discover their genes have decided to wipe out their memory. In reality, that only happens if something drastic changes in your system. The gene needs to express itself differently, and the only way to express something differently is to have a trigger. A great example is elephants. They have multiple copies of the APOE4 gene, which is related to neurological disorders and the one most people hope they don't have when they look at their genetic reports. Elephants are known for having the best memories and don't get Alzheimer's.[40] They have the gene, but it isn't expressed because whatever they do—their lifestyle—keeps that from happening.

The same rule applies to us. If we can take the trigger away, it doesn't matter what gene we have; the gene becomes immaterial. All that matters is being aware of the trigger and getting ahead of it.

And so, if you've been worried about your health because your grandfather had a heart attack at 72, and you're concerned the same might happen to you, you can relax a bit. It's not guaranteed. However, it is important to avoid the triggers associated with the gene (if you have inherited it).

What triggers our genes is heavily influenced by the activity of the microbes inside our gut, mouth, and all over us. But this is also very good news. Our daily choices impact our health and are *under our control.* If you figure out how to avoid the trigger that turns on the offending gene, you have a chance at avoiding its ill effects. This is why understanding RNA is extremely important. So, let me explain it.

Understanding RNA

Here is my layman's way of understanding and explaining RNA to folks outside of scientific circles. Every cell in your body has identical DNA. If you take a cell sample from your skin, elbows, or hair follicles, each contains the same DNA. It doesn't matter what tissue you take. So, why don't we have eyes growing on our fingers or nails sprouting from our hips? Because different genes are expressed in different parts of the body.

To better understand gene expression, think of the process like a cook making a recipe from a cookbook. DNA, made up of genes, contains instructions (the recipe). RNA acts as the cook that reads these instructions to make a "dish," which is a protein. The resulting protein is a complex molecule that can fold into various shapes and perform many functions, such as building structures, speeding up chemical reactions, and transporting molecules.[41] Abnormal (excessive or insufficient) protein production from this process is what causes disease states. So, understanding and managing gene expression is key to preventing age-related decline and illness.

There is this idea that we are born with our health destiny pre-written. But our genes are not our destiny. Aging and disease are caused by abnormal gene expression, which is triggered by various factors such as diet, toxins, and the environment. Nutrients from food, harmful substances, and environmental conditions like temperature and light can all influence which genes are turned on or off. Hormones, physical activity, and stress also play significant roles in regulating gene expression, allowing cells to adapt and respond to their surroundings and internal signals.

All of us live such different lifestyles with different medical histories, in different locations, with different partners and friends and pets. Combined with the uniqueness of our microbial communities, we need to be able to monitor changes to our body in order to know how to modulate them for the benefit of the person. Gene expression allows for personalization and dynamic recommendations, solutions, and products.

Understanding these triggers, how they affect each individual uniquely, and learning how to get ahead of them became a critical mission in my new venture. Once my team and I figured this out, we had a path forward. We would digitize the human body. And thus, it became the next focus in our pursuit.

The Mindshift Shift

If you take one insight from this chapter, let it be this...

Your DNA is not your destiny. Gene expression (RNA) determines your state of health.

RNA is a readout of your DNA and is used to build important components the body needs to function. If RNA messages get muddled, genes for disease may be abnormally expressed, which can lead to disease.

You have control over your microbial and human gene expression. It comes down to what you do—your diet and your lifestyle.

Key Insights

- Why This? Why Now? Why Me? is my three-question process for deciding if it makes sense to pursue a mission in life or business.
- A moonshot is a goal most people believe is impossible to achieve.
- A symbolic moonshot is a type of moonshot that's about improving life for a billion people. It's any massive goal that reshapes societal narratives.
- Aging and illness are two of the world's greatest epidemics and problems. It's also a major paradox.

Each year, the U.S. spends trillions on healthcare, and the wellness economy continues to grow. Yet, people are developing more chronic diseases and health conditions at younger ages.

- We have never experienced a time like this with the acceleration and convergence of technologies. We have more tools than ever to create superior health innovations that are affordable and accessible.

- Technological growth is exponential. Computing processing power continues to speed up. Each iteration of a tool can be used to build the next version, which is why tools get faster and cheaper over time.

- Many technologies are reshaping health and wellness. With new advances, it is possible to build more personalized solutions that provide deeper insights.

- When scientists cracked the code on the Human Genome, they learned that the human body has approximately 23,000 genes. Shortly after, DNA technologies and products grew in popularity.

- When the human body changes, its DNA stays the same. Even when we're sick.

- Gene expression determines our state of health. RNA reads our DNA and uses it to build proteins that cells need to function. Excessive protein production results in disease and aging.

- To build a solution, the team at Viome focused on digitizing the human body so we could understand the triggers that lead to gene expression and disease and aging and create solutions to prevent that from happening.

CHAPTER 3
DIGITIZING THE HUMAN BODY

*Our human bodies are miracles, not because they
defy laws of nature, but precisely because they
obey them.*

— Harold S. Kushner, American Author

I needed experts to guide me in unlocking the secrets
of human health and longevity. To find them, I adopted
a "Shark Tank" approach. You might be familiar with
the popular reality television show featuring aspiring
entrepreneurs who pitch their business ideas or products to a panel of investors called "sharks." Instead of
entrepreneurs, I searched for scientists working on technologies that might help me bootstrap my moonshot.

I visited the NASA centers in Pasadena, AMES, Houston, and Cape Canaveral. Then I traveled to all the top universities from Stanford, MIT, and Duke, to Lawrence Berkeley. I asked each scientist I met to do a "Shark Tank"-style presentation about their work for me where they pitch their ideas. This approach helped me understand how their technologies could address the problems I was focused on, and it led me to Los Alamos National Lab (LANL), where I finally found what I needed.

For the unacquainted, Los Alamos is where the U.S. government built the first atomic bombs used during World War II. It's the primary nuclear weapons research facility in the United States. In other words, if there is one place where they know about security, it's LANL. At LANL, I met Dr. Momo Vuyisich, a leading systems biologist working in biodefense at the time.

The U.S. government was concerned that malicious actors might one day develop technologies capable of making people sick. Momo's role was to create government-funded technology to counter these potential threats. In the event that a biological threat was detected, an antidote would be crucial to defend against it. The solution was to develop a technology that could classify every microorganism in the body, determine their functions, and identify how to counteract any disease-causing behavior they might exhibit in individuals. In other words, they were conducting gene expression (RNA) analysis of all the microbes in the human body, as well as analyzing gene expression for each one.

During his presentation, Momo was somewhat vague out of necessity because the project he was working on was top secret. Even with his limited description, I suspected that his work could be the solution I needed. If this technology had the power to analyze this level of detail about the microbiome, it could also be used to analyze the unique response of each individual's microbiome to other things, like nutrition.

After several trips and thorough discussions, I eventually realized that his technology was indeed what I was looking for. The next step was to license it and build a team to implement it, which took another six months. The final challenge was to convince him to leave his secure, federally guaranteed job and join my start-up company.

I later learned that Momo was diagnosed with an idiopathic autoimmune disease in his twenties. Idiopathic means no one can figure out the cause. The only solution he was given was to prime his system with anti-inflammatories. He took very strong drugs for many years, but he continued to deteriorate, suffering low-grade inflammation, joint and soft tissue pain, and many other symptoms. As he worked on his Ph.D. in chemistry, he learned that our bodies are simply sacks of chemicals that process tens of thousands of chemical reactions. When one of them goes out of whack, so does our health. This was one of the reasons why he was motivated to join the start-up and help me solve this problem.

Having Momo on board solved the first piece of the puzzle, which was to digitize the human body. Now I needed someone who could process massive amounts of data and analyze it using cutting-edge AI to make sense of what was happening inside the body at the onset and during the progression of all the chronic diseases, cancer, and aging.

Soon after I hired Momo, I got a call from Guruduth "Guru" Banavar, then the head of research at IBM Watson. Guru is one of the world leaders in artificial intelligence. He had spent twenty years working on the first computer system to answer questions posed in natural language. You might recall that IBM Watson, a supercomputer, made headlines when it beat experts on *Jeopardy!* in 2011. A computer took home the first-place prize of $1 million. Guru told me that if we knew what to look for in the human body, he could build a technology solution to analyze the data.

He ended up joining Viome as our head of AI and Chief Technology Officer (CTO) to build Vie, our AI platform designed to digitize, decode, and decipher microbial activity in the human body. To get there, Guru needed critical biological data, and I already had Momo on board to provide him with the data he needed.

At that point, we had what we needed to launch Viome, the first company in the world focused on making aging and illness a choice. The hope was to give people the tools and information they needed to be in control of their health. When you have the data and the plan you need to improve your health, you get to decide what steps to take next, and that makes your health choices straightforward.

Since 2016, many of the world's best scientists, doctors, and nutritionists have joined our mission. Together, we have been on a remarkable journey of scientific discovery to get to the root of what makes people age and get sick so we can develop innovative, personalized solutions and life-saving tests to get ahead of it.

We truly live in the most amazing time in human history. We have more information and sophisticated technological tools than ever before. When we started, we had yet to learn how to get to where we are today. We began with an audacious goal and questions like: *What makes us sick? Why do we even get sick? Why do some people live a healthy life into their nineties while others at 67 can barely walk? We're all human, yet there are so many variations between us. So, what's the difference?* It's not like there's programming in the human body that triggers a disease when you hit a certain age, *'Happy birthday, you're 50. It's time for diabetes!'*

Given the technological advances of the time and those coming on the horizon, we knew it would be possible to create a solution to avoid aging and illness. We also understood that science is ever-evolving, constantly bringing new insights to light and changing the course of history with new variables. The key to building a successful company is the ability to pivot, build upon what you know, be ready and open to learn what you don't, and always consider what's out there to help you reach your goal faster. Staying focused on our mission while remaining adaptable has been crucial in navigating this journey and advancing toward our vision.

Making aging and illness optional was simply a matter of finding the right experts to make my equation below a reality.

$$\frac{Biological}{Intelligence} + \frac{Human}{Intelligence} \times \frac{Artificial}{Intelligence} = \frac{Precision}{Health}$$

We needed these three elements to come together. And remarkably, that is just what happened.

This equation is the basis of our success as a company at the forefront of precision health, where we can make decisions based on our own bodies' data, even as it evolves over time. Throughout this book, you will learn how critical these three elements are to the future of health and longevity. We and others use them every day to demystify the human body and learn how to keep it healthy.

Once I had the core team in place, we wondered, *What if we could digitize the human body and make it like an Airbus A380?*

A Proactive Approach to Health: Continuous Monitoring and Maintenance

The Airbus A380 is a mechanical marvel. It is the most sophisticated plane and one of the most complicated machines humans have ever built. These massive double-decker planes carry 450 people and fly up to 640 miles per hour. As the world's largest passenger aircraft, the superjumbo, as it is called, is engineered with the most modern materials to reduce weight and increase fuel efficiency. Built with over 100,000 miles of wire, quadruple redundant systems for hydraulics, and the most sophisticated pressurization software, intricate engineering ensures its safety, structural integrity, and efficiency.[42]

Hundreds of these planes have taken to the air and flown for millions of hours. To this day, not once has there been a fatal Airbus A380 accident.[43] While it's easy to brush that off and think, "It's a plane. Who cares?" The Airbus A380 has been ingeniously engineered.

Ensuring seamless integration and functionality of its engines, avionics, hydraulics, and fuel systems is a significant engineering challenge. Engineers designing the Airbus A380 must consider the entire system to ensure that each component, no matter how small, functions perfectly within the whole. The design of each part, from the tiniest wire to the largest engine, is informed by an understanding of its role within the larger system. This holistic approach is essential for achieving the high levels of safety, efficiency, and performance required for such a complex machine.

We learned that the engineers maintaining the Airbus A380 know everything about it. The plane is built with 100,000 sensors. When a sensor sends an alert because there's an issue, it's repaired immediately. The experts who monitor these plans are also extensively trained. They know how long each part will last and when one might wear out. And they replace everything well in advance. It's an approach of continuous monitoring and maintenance.[44] And it's what Viome is doing for the human body.

Let's put this into perspective. If Airbus A380 engineers took a similar approach to what we do in genetics today, it would look very different. Before takeoff, an expert might analyze the plane and see it has a 9 percent chance of three accidents in the next twenty five years. What would you do if you were an A380 passenger and heard those numbers? Likely, you'd do nothing. There's a potential for an accident, not a certainty that it will happen.

As I mentioned before, DNA analysis gives us the potential in a person for a particular illness or disease. Just because you have a gene for cancer doesn't mean you will get it. So, instead of DNA analysis, we focus on

71

gene expression, and our technology allows us to analyze and interpret RNA. And our ultimate focus has been to digitize the human body so we can monitor critical factors that lead to illness and get ahead of it, just like the Airbus A380 engineers do with the aircraft to avoid catastrophic crashes.

We discovered that by creating a digital template for our biology, we could constantly monitor various parts of the body and adjust them to ensure optimal health. This is the foundation of our approach at Viome. We don't just monitor the genetic potential for disease; we also track gene expression, which signals the onset and progression of disease, and determine how we can modulate it using nutrition.

This information is derived from processing samples of saliva, blood, and stool from at-home collection kits. From these samples, we can extract billions of data points. By comparison, when a doctor orders a lipid panel, the lab can only extract a few data points from that test. You can imagine how billions of data points provide a much more comprehensive picture than just a few. And this is only the beginning. We can also analyze the data to determine if a gene is over- or under-expressing.

Getting to this point was an incredibly complex journey. Our first step in digitizing the human body was to understand all the conditions that lead to a dysfunctional state.

Now imagine how challenging that is, too! The human body is extremely complex. It's why the field of biology is as well. Unlike other fields of science, so many variables impact the body where simple cause-and-effect principles are nearly impossible. While a chemist can precisely measure temperature increases in a reaction, and physicists can calculate force, it's much more complicated for a biologist. Living entities are the most complex systems in existence. It is excessively difficult and time-consuming to perform detailed calculations on biological systems.[45]

To grasp the complexity of the process, consider that a single cell contains a vast array of molecules intricately arranged in a tiny space. These molecules engage in countless biochemical reactions driven by enzymes. Additionally, the cell is influenced by external factors such as drugs, hormones, or changes in nutritional availability. This introduces us to systems biology, which has been central to our research.[46]

At Viome, we take a systems biology approach because it is more sophisticated and accurate than traditional biology. Traditional biology focuses on reductionism, breaking down an object into its components. In contrast, systems biology embraces holism, understanding that parts of a whole are interconnected and cannot exist or be fully understood independently.[47]

For instance, if you were a patient seeing a systems biologist physician about a mood issue, say depression, they would not simply immediately treat your symptoms with a drug. They would do an exploration to get to the root, which would consider a variety of environmental, social, and biological factors. For example, they might look at data from cells and molecules, and look at organ function and brain regions. They would integrate this information with factors that consider your family genetic and relationship dynamics, community, and what you might be exposed to based on where you live. This is a very different approach than how our current healthcare system is structured, where the body is treated in individual subparts (urology, cardiology, dermatology, etc.).

Since system biology integrates many scientific disciplines—from traditional biology to computer science, engineering, bioinformatics, physics, and more—it requires massive amounts of data. Systems biologists use complex mathematical modeling to calculate interactions of components to predict a system's activity. Before AI, this wasn't easy. The human mind can't keep track of so many processes in parallel. However, AI-powered computers can.

Using AI machine learning systems allows us to examine many complex ecosystems that are always changing—from our diet to processes in our bodies to the environments we live in. To understand our health, we need to analyze quadrillions of data points. To help you visualize that giant number, one quadrillion is approximately the number of gallons of water that flow over Niagara Falls in 210 years.[48]

So, by using systems biology and applying AI to digitize the human body, we can process massive amounts of data, giving us insights into our deepest inner workings, which is what we needed to get ahead of aging and disease.

Your Body Is a Universe

As a young boy growing up in rural India, most of what I knew of the world was what I could see around me. But each night, I would gaze at the Moon and stars, very much taken by the celestial marvel that hung in the sky. To me, it was a beacon of possibility.

I realized that even the richest person in the world had the same access to the Moon as me. It was impossibly far away, but it held a special attraction that allowed me to dream beyond my village and country. There are trillions of stars in our Universe; what we see is just a minuscule part of our mysterious cosmos.

Today, my perspective has evolved. While I still marvel at what is in the sky, from the stars to planets, I see the world as a minute and intricate network of trillions of microbes.

Our bodies are covered in microscopic entities, invisible to the naked eye that are as complex and fascinating as the Moon, planets, and stars that once captivated my imagination as a boy. Just as the cosmos consists of galaxies and solar systems within them, our bodies consist of a human microbiome which is the collection of all microbes that reside on or within us. We have microbes living in our human tissues and biofluids and they live in colonies that populate different areas of our bodies. There is a microbiome in our gut, in our mouths, on our skin, in our respiratory tracts, in our reproductive organs, and even in our blood.

We are an ever-changing, complex host to these tiny organisms. Our microbiome is also extremely dynamic. We share and receive microorganisms from other humans through touch, intimacy, and everyday interaction. We also interact with the Earth's microbiome, giving and receiving microbes via the air we breathe, the places we go, and the creatures we interact with.

To help people understand our deep, symbiotic relationship with this veritable cosmos of microbes, I often tell a story that helps explain how it all came to be.

—

The Greatest Story of Creation Never Told: An Alternate Tongue-in-Cheek Take on Reality

Three and half billion years ago, hoards of single-celled beasties occupied the planet. Life was hard for these tiny creatures. They had to forage for their food. The environment was harsh, and it took them ages to travel short distances. Over the millennia, they became disgruntled with their lot in life. Having reached their limit, they convened a special council to plot a new course.

The most intelligent microbe of all concocted a plan.

He said: "My fellow microbes, I have a solution to all our problems. We will build an animal, a home where we can live and thrive forever."

After a bit of trial and error with reptiles, fish, and gorillas, the microbes finally perfected their formula to make humans. Inside humans, the microscopic beasties would be safe, and all their needs would be met. They would receive food from their human hosts. Humans would also be a great vessel to travel the world. In their journeys they would spread the microbes around so they could build new communities, interact with other microbes, and grow their population. In exchange, they would keep humans healthy.

As humans evolved, they grew bigger brains and became more advanced. About 200 million years ago, they grew a brain region called the neocortex, which allowed them to have advanced thinking. The

microorganisms started to worry and became para-
noid. They thought that the new Intelligence is going to
take over the world! Just like some humans today are
afraid of AI, these microbes were worried about their
existence.

Luckily, they had thought ahead. Most microbes live in
the human gut, and there is a direct connection from
the gut to the brain called the "vagus" nerve. Microbes
thought the name we humans gave was ironic because,
unlike Las Vegas, where the saying goes that what
happens in Vegas stays in Vegas, what happens in the
gut goes everywhere, and our whole body is impacted.
Through the vagus nerve, microbes in our gut are able to
make us crave the food they want and they can control
many of the functions of our brain with the neurotrans-
mitters they produce. Ninety percent of all serotonin, a
biochemical that makes us feel good, is produced in our
gut. Additionally, inside each human cell are mitochondria, which supply all the energy to the human body.
These mitochondria are actually microbes that became
part of our human cells in a symbiotic relationship. They
have the same microbial communication mechanism, so
our microbes are able to easily communicate with them,
changing their behavior and adjusting the energy they
produce.

—

It's a silly story, and though it might seem ridiculous
that microorganisms are so sophisticated that they could
organize, plot their survival, and build humans, it might
just be closer to the truth than other creation tales.

Over three billion years ago, tiny molecules called amino acids formed DNA, the blueprint for all living things. It allowed simple cells to develop and evolve into more complex creatures. Scientists now understand that the earliest life forms were microscopic organisms. Early microbes left traces in rocks 3.7 billion years ago.[49] We know this because scientists have found evidence of the same carbon molecules in all living entities. So, microbes were on Earth long before the earliest humans, which we've tracked back to about six million years. Modern humans—us—only evolved about 200,000 years ago.[50]

Scientists have only just begun to understand this symbiotic relationship with microbes. In recent decades, they discovered that the microorganisms in our bodies control almost everything. How harmoniously we live with them strongly determines our health and biological age. We have about 40 trillion microbes inside us.[51] The exact number varies widely among individuals based on diet, oral hygiene, and overall health. However, as a general rule, our bodies have as many microbial cells as human cells.

In essence, *they are us, and we are them.*

We have microorganisms in our gut that control our brain's amygdala and prefrontal cortex. Others control our energy by impacting the mitochondria in each cell, and they dictate our biological age. Here, you'll also see how a diverse microbiome has been linked to longevity. The microbiome has also been linked to almost every minor condition and chronic disease, including weight gain, digestive problems, and skin issues. It is also linked to greater issues like cancer, heart disease, and brain conditions like anxiety, depression, and Alzheimer's.

But it's not only what's in us that matters. There are microbes in everything around us, and as we navigate the world and interact with it, our microbial makeup changes, too.

Without microbes, life on planet Earth would die. The Earth contains a hugely diverse microbial com-

There are microbes in everything around us, and as we navigate the world and interact with it, our microbial makeup changes, too

munity. They live in the air and the dirt. There are millions of microbes in a single teaspoon of soil. Our oceans and freshwater are packed with microbial life, too. Ninety percent of the mass of all living things in the ocean is from microbes. Microorganisms even live in extreme temperatures, from the freezing waters of the glacial lakes to boiling hydrothermal vents. They live on plants and the bodies of animals.[52]

We now understand that the human microbiome impacts every area of our health, from digestion to immunity to cellular health. It's why recently, there's been a blow up of microbiome and gut-related documentaries, books, and courses on all the major platforms. Before I launched Viome, I saw this wave coming.

Every time I start a company, I become an information junkie and I search and filter for critical information. I set up my news feeds to sift through everything on health and wellness, and the bookmarks on my computer contain links to the latest research journals. I also call friends who are experts in the business to get an industry pulse.

As I shared earlier, in 2016, I noticed that research on the microbiome was piling up. At first, there were tens, then hundreds, and eventually thousands of published papers. I realized microbiome science and solutions would be mainstream in three to five years. With thousands of papers linking microbiome to health and aging,

I could tell it was a growing area. Within three years, I figured everyone would be talking about microbiology, and sure enough, that's what happened. People say I had a crystal ball. But I was simply a motivated entrepreneur looking for a way to avoid accelerated aging and chronic disease.

So, that is where our attention as a company was drawn. We would use our technology to understand the human microbiome and we had an inkling that it would reveal the secret to lifelong health. It wasn't long until we realized we were right.

The Forgotten Organ

Scientists have known about the microbes living in and on our bodies since the 17th century. However, as you already learned, the microbiome didn't become a major focus until the human genome was sequenced in the early 2000s.

Nevertheless, the first connection was made way back in 1670 by a clever Dutch scientist who used handcrafted microscopes to observe and describe the first microorganisms. Back then, he called them "animalcules," which might be a better word given their level of sophistication.[53] This groundbreaking observation marked the first awareness of microscopic life forms. Then, over time, scientists learned that microbes colonize the body and co-exist with us as lifelong partners, which led to germ theory in the 19th century.[54]

During that time, more scientists made the connection between microorganisms and disease. Unfortunately, as we'll explore later, this has led to some misperceptions about microbes. It also led to positive medical innovations, like antibiotics, a scientific wonder that changed the course of medicine and human health. However, antibiotics have a downside, too. Excessive use of them has become a major health threat (more on this soon). Still, germ theory was pivotal in our understanding of microbes and human health.

Through the 20th century, there were even more advances in microbiology. Then, in the last few decades, our understanding of the human microbiome expanded exponentially thanks to the advent of advanced genomic and computational technologies. Scientists mapped the human genome in the late 1990s, and the work led to the startling revelation that simple house plants had more genes than we did. But, as you learned, it all made sense when they learned about microbes. If we look at the genes of the approximately 40 trillion microbes in and on our bodies, we see that they outnumber our genes by about 100 to 1.[55] The human microbiome is as important as our heart, liver, brain, and all the other vital organs that keep us alive.

Once this connection was made in the early 2000s, deeper attention and a flurry of further scientific exploration followed. Today, microbiologists and scientific teams around the world are publishing new research papers relating to the microbiome with accelerating frequency. Yet, there is still much to discover about how the little organisms impact our health. We continue to ask questions like: Why don't they kill us? Why don't we kill them? What forces maintain equilibrium among the populations of these tiny bugs? How do individuals differ from one another microbiologically? And most importantly, how can we manipulate microbes to fight or avoid disease altogether?

What we do know is they are not evil parasites. We rely on them. For example, some help us digest certain foods, like fiber. The human body cannot digest it without them. They also release short-chain fatty acids, which our body needs to stay healthy. Many vitamins our body needs, like Vitamins B, C, and K, are also produced by microorganisms.[56] So when we feed them, they feed us. Therefore, what we feed them is important.

So, for our team, we needed to understand how that happens. It led to more questions like: How do we get microbes? How do they function? And how do we nurture them so they keep us healthy?

Me, Microbes, and I

Suppose we took a group of one hundred people from the same location and looked at each of their microbiomes under a microscope. We would find that no person has the same microbial makeup. Certain people might have somewhat similar microbes because they live in the same geographic region. However, every individual has a one-of-a-kind community that we each get as we enter the world, because our mothers give us our first microbes.[57] Microorganisms coat a newborn's skin as it journeys through the birth canal during delivery. Later, more microbes are transferred through breast milk. We collect more still when our parents kiss, touch, and coo over us.[58] Since we all acquire our first microbes from Mom, imagine how important it is for her to be healthy.

Anyone reading this who was born by Cesarean Section (C-Section) or had one will wonder what happens. We're now learning that C-Sections may negatively impact health.[59] Later in this chapter, we'll look at this more closely. But for now, this doesn't mean we shouldn't use these important life-saving medical innovations. It's more about exercising caution and understanding negative effects and how to counteract them.

Our first exposure to microbes supports the growth and development of our digestive and nervous systems. Our immune system also learns from microbes. It starts to understand what the body should recognize as a friend or foe. Then, throughout our lives, we're exposed to factors that continue to shape our microbiomes. That includes the environment we grow up in—whether urban or rural—the presence of pets and other animals, and our dietary habits. Other impacts include exposure to environmental toxins like fungicides, herbicides, and pesticides. Medications disrupt the microbiome, too. Then there are the things we do, like exercise, sleep, work, and hobbies. Even stress has an impact.[60]

Some microbes are with us forever. Think of them like the barnacles attached to whales, hitching a ride for life. Other microbes are only visitors. They stick around for weeks, months, or years. We constantly undergo microbial changes based on many variables, from our environment to diet and connection with others. These variables can be either helpful for our health or increase our risk of sickness and decline due to aging.

Understanding how our microbes are linked to our health is extremely complex. Therefore, scientists have taken the most logical route to unpack the mystery of the human microbiome. They started with the most densely populated regions of the body that are also the most easily accessible. The gut falls into both categories, so most microbiome research has largely focused on it.[61]

The mouth has been researchers' second greatest area of focus, given the high density of organisms found there and the ease of accessibility—no need for needles or probes. You just need to say "ahhh" to access a sample. On average, it's estimated that the mouth contains more than 400 microbial species, with the total number of cells in the billions.[62]

Another area that has drawn much attention is the human genital regions and the urinary tract. There has been more emphasis on understanding women because they give birth. Additionally, there are microbial communities in the skin and respiratory tract, and studies have been conducted on the microbial connection to the human immune system.[63]

Figure 3.1—Microbiomes of the Human Body

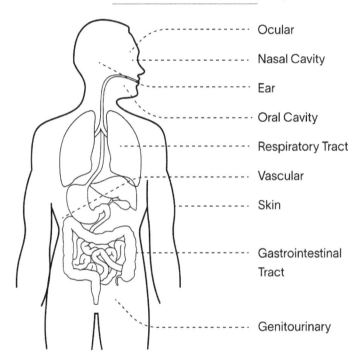

Microbiomes of the Human Body

Ocular

Nasal Cavity

Ear

Oral Cavity

Respiratory Tract

Vascular

Skin

Gastrointestinal
Tract

Genitourinary

*The various microbiomes of the body that collectively are
referred to as the human microbiome.*

Each community of microbes is like a neighbor-
hood in a city, and some areas of the body are more
densely populated. The gut is like Manhattan in New
York City. It has the highest population density with
over 70,000 people per square mile, even though it's
geographically the smallest region. The mouth's microbiome might be Brooklyn, the second densely packed

area. In contrast, some regions have microbes living further apart, like Staten Island. It would be more like the skin's microbiome.

Diverse microorganisms, like city inhabitants, also occupy every community of the body. Take Manhattan's diverse demography. Its inhabitants are a mixture of Caucasian, Hispanic, African American, Asian, and multiracial people. Similarly, the body has diverse communities of microbes in each region. In each ecosystem, these microorganisms interact, making and forming biofilms that protect each other. How each species works together causes us to remain or get sick. Each microbial community influences how systems run in every body area, including digestion, energy, sleep, cognition, mood, immune, oral, and metabolic health.

Now think of how we describe ethnic groups, bucketing very different groups into one. We often do the same with microbes, though each one is unique, like people. For instance, when people use the term Indian, they could be speaking about the Indo-Aryans from North, Central, and West, the Dravidians from South, the Austroasiatic, and so on. The same is true of microbes. Each diverse microbiota community is a collection of tiny creatures that fall under four key classifications: 1) bacteria, 2) viruses and bacteriophages, 3) fungi, and 4) archaea.[64] For geeks like me who like to go deeper into the science, you can learn more about each type at TheYouthFormula.com

To complicate the situation further, each microbe is like a person with distinct beliefs, values, and functions. Our cultural backgrounds, day-to-day environments, and the people around us shape us. They inform what we do, and microbes are similarly differentiated. Like humans, where no person is entirely good or bad, the same applies to microorganisms. They have both good and bad functions.

In a healthy body, different microbes peacefully coexist. But if there's a disruption in this balance caused by infections, specific diets, or prolonged use of certain medications like antibiotics, it causes disease.

Healthspan is a Game of Dodgeball Dysbiosis

If you search the web for any chronic health condition, from obesity to Alzheimer's to heart disease, along with "microbiome," you'll find intriguing research linking the microbiome to almost every health problem, acute to chronic.

The bottom line of every health condition and disease is that we want to avoid *dysbiosis*.

Dysbiosis is science-speak for a condition in which the microbes in our body do not coexist peacefully.[65] Instead, they are in conflict. To simplify this concept, let's go back to our New York City analogy. Dysbiosis is akin to a scenario where a group of New Yorkers are arguing over who gets the last black-and-white cookie at a coffee shop.

To cover every study on this topic in depth would fill a book, and it can make for dry reading if we were to regurgitate every technical detail here, especially if they are irrelevant to you. And so we won't cover studies like this one from 2020: *Acute appendicitis is associated with appendiceal microbiome changes, including elevated Campylobacter jejuni levels.* You get the idea, right?

Nevertheless, it's essential to highlight the most significant discoveries in this area. Researchers have found surprising connections, such as the similarity between gut and brain plaques, how weight gain is linked to antibiotics in our food and the identification of certain microbes as cancer-causing agents.

Below, I've listed the headlines of some of the most groundbreaking studies that have captured my team's attention and that of the global community. You can find the studies relevant to you at TheYouthFormula.com. There, we've summarized the key findings in a digestible manner.

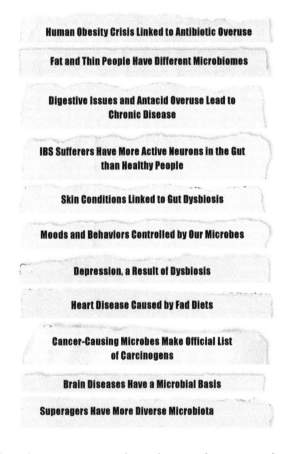

Human Obesity Crisis Linked to Antibiotic Overuse

Fat and Thin People Have Different Microbiomes

Digestive Issues and Antacid Overuse Lead to Chronic Disease

IBS Sufferers Have More Active Neurons in the Gut than Healthy People

Skin Conditions Linked to Gut Dysbiosis

Moods and Behaviors Controlled by Our Microbes

Depression, a Result of Dysbiosis

Heart Disease Caused by Fad Diets

Cancer-Causing Microbes Make Official List of Carcinogens

Brain Diseases Have a Microbial Basis

Superagers Have More Diverse Microbiota

For those interested in diving deeper, we've also compiled a comprehensive library of journals. We encourage anyone with a specific health issue to consult TheYouthFormula.com for further insights.

As you can see, the microbiome is connected to numerous diseases. This raises a crucial question: What is happening to us that's leading to microbial health imbalances in the majority of people? And if that's the case, what steps can we take to avoid the problem?

What's Causing Dysbiosis?

As I wrote earlier, my dad's shortened lifespan was likely a result of his modern lifestyle. He is not unique. The problems that likely caused his illnesses and shortened life are affecting us all.

We are becoming sicker and aging faster because our modern lifestyle puts pressure on the microbes living in and around us. This imbalance is caused by factors such as constant stress, lack of exercise, and insufficient sleep. There are seven major scenarios we know cause trauma for microbes today that are worth examining. They are:

1. Antibiotics overuse in humans
2. Cesarean Sections
3. Pesticides in farming
4. Antibiotics in livestock
5. Processed food
6. Microbial extinction

Now, I realize this list is going to occur as a lot of doom and gloom. My intention is not to scare you, just to lay out what we as humans are facing. We can't address problems until we define what they are, and I want you to understand the challenges we are all up against.

Let's start with antimicrobial resistance, a topic not enough people know about.

Antibiotics Overuse in Humans

While antibiotics are useful because they kill dangerous bacterial infections, their overuse is an equal threat. Over time, some bacteria can develop a resistance to antibiotics, leading to infections that are harder to treat and that can spread more easily.[66]

An antibiotics overuse crisis could lead to higher healthcare costs, reduced productivity, and increased poverty, severely impacting global economic stability. It also threatens to undermine the foundations of modern medicine, possibly ushering in a post-antibiotic era where current treatments become obsolete.[67]

Addressing this issue requires a unified global effort to promote preventative measures among healthcare providers, farmers, and veterinarians, aiming to reduce infections and optimize the use of antimicrobial drugs.

Cesarean Sections

A Cesarean Section is a crucial surgical procedure where a baby is removed from its mother via an incision in her belly. It is usually administered as an emergency procedure when a baby can't transit through a mother's birth canal.

C-Sections save the lives of both mothers and babies. However, some experts argue that they are performed more often than necessary, which could lead to long-term health issues for babies delivered this way. A C-Section can impact a baby's microbiome negatively and cause health issues for a child as they grow because they do not pick up vital microorganisms as they are born.[68]

The good news is experiments are currently under-way where cells from the mother's vagina are collected and applied to the baby following a C-Section delivery. In the near future, it's likely we will see new solutions emerge to restore microbial communities at the beginning of a person's life.[69]

Antibiotics in Livestock

Antibiotics are commonly given to many livestock animals, like cows, pigs, and turkeys, so they gain weight.[70] Plump and juicy meat is also highly appealing. However, now there are concerns and studies showing the widespread negative effects of this method of farming. The use of antibiotics in this manner is fostering concern about the development of antibiotic resistance and health concerns like obesity in humans.

Industrialized animal husbandry is also responsible for the rise in zoonotic diseases, where pathogens jump between animals and people. COVID-19 is a good example where an animal virus jumped to a human in a market in Wuhan, China, and resulted in a pandemic.[71]

With growing concerns about the way meat is pro-duced, it might make sense to switch to a vegetarian or plant-based lifestyle. However, that's not the whole solu-tion because modern food-growing techniques have also changed the microbial density of our vegetables and fruits.

Pesticides in Farming

Since the 1950s, artificial fertilizers, chemical bug killers, and agriscience have been used in food production to make it more commercially appealing, abundant, and, in some cases, more affordable.[72] We have more ability than ever to make perfect-looking food with genetically modified technologies and pesticides. However, these innovations impact our foods' quality and nutritional value. The food we grow today is less nutrient-dense than it was decades ago, and soil depletion is one of the biggest causes. Modern intensive agricultural methods also strip nutrients from the soil that we use.[73]

Numerous studies published in the late 1980s and early 2000s found a major decline in the nutrient density of up to 43 vegetables and fruits in various countries. These studies found a range of 21-37 percent decline in the nutritional value of various crops. The crops had less calcium, phosphorus, protein, iron, riboflavin (Vitamin B2), and Vitamin C. Research suggests that declining nutritional content is connected to modern agricultural practices designed to improve growth and appearance and reduce pests.[74]

When we use toxic agents to grow our food, it affects our bodies. The manure used by farmers also becomes less microbial-dense. Agriculture practices are leading to more chemicals, antibiotics, and growth hormones in our water, posing risks to us and aquatic ecosystems. The way we treat our environments has major implications that impact us later.

So, is avoiding farmed and animal foods a solution? What could we eat instead? We could engineer better foods or process them, but that has issues, too.

Processed Foods

The statistical links between processed foods and disease in the U.S. and the world are a subject of ongoing research. While it is challenging to establish direct causation between processed foods and specific diseases, there is a growing body of evidence.

Many studies have shown a positive association between the consumption of ultra-processed foods and the risk of obesity and weight gain. We know that highly processed foods, with added sugars, unhealthy fats, and empty calories, can contribute to overeating and an increased risk of obesity-related diseases, such as type 2 diabetes and cardiovascular diseases, including hypertension, coronary artery disease, and stroke.[75]

Additionally, processed meats, like bacon and hot dogs, have been classified as carcinogens, indicating they are known to cause cancer.[76] Processed foods with high levels of preservatives and additives may also be associated with increased cancer risk, but more research is needed.

What is clear, however, is that processed foods have less nutritional value and potentially disruptive microbial effects. Consuming highly processed foods may decrease the intake of naturally occurring microbes.

Yet, the microbiome is not just influenced by our diet. Our bodies interact with a dynamic and ever-changing environment where the activities we engage in and the places we visit also affect our internal ecosystem.

Microbial Extinction

The Earth's microbiome is a critical life-support system for our planet. Microorganisms serve many functions in planetary life. They support the decomposition of organic matter and play a role in maintaining the key cycles of life, including the production of carbon, hydrogen, nitrogen, oxygen, phosphorus, and sulfur. But our planet is becoming less microbial-dense because we've industrialized the natural world. According to scientists, every time we lose a species of animal or plant that goes extinct, so do many microbes.[77]

Many studies have proven this. For instance, research conducted in the Netherlands found that many fungi are going extinct. Similar research was conducted in Germany. The same piece of German woodland was studied 3500 times between 1950 and 1985, where major declines in fungal species were recorded.[78]

Efforts are also underway to understand the human microbiome by evaluating ancestral remains. One study analyzed feces collected from caves in the U.S. and Mexico. The data was used to reconstruct and understand the microbial composition of our human ancestors. The DNA was analyzed using modern gene technology to examine the microbial makeup of 181 samples between 1000-2000 years old. Genetic material from early humans was compared with the gut microbiome of modern people. The scientists found that early remains contained 39 percent microbial species that had not been seen before, showing that extinction is happening in us, too.[79]

Today, most people also spend more time indoors, where microbial diversity is generally lower than in outdoor environments. Reduced exposure to natural ecosystems and outdoor activities limits our contact with diverse microbial communities. So, let's all get outside. No need to be afraid of germs. As you'll see, that can be a problem too.

Ill-Conceived Germophobia

There was once a collectively held notion that health equates to germ-free bodies. The belief that good health results from germ avoidance is widespread, from childhood taunts about "cooties"' to the overuse of cleaning chemicals.

A case in point was the COVID-19 pandemic, during which hand sanitizer sales spiked 600 percent.[80] Although usage has lessened since then, it is still high compared to pre-COVID times. Higher usage is understandable given the threat at the time, but it is potentially harmful in the long term.

Spiking public fear after health crises is normal. Media, advertisers, and politicians often exploit these fears for profit, audience growth, and votes, shaping new cultural health norms. We've seen this pattern repeatedly, from the 1918 flu pandemic, which led to heightened germaphobia and public health education, to the post-World War II era, which saw the rise of toothbrushing with fluoride toothpaste. Similarly, recent global warming concerns have significantly increased sunscreen use, driven by heightened awareness of skin cancer risks. While these responses to threats lead to new norms and innovations, they also reveal unintended consequences.[81]

The widespread use of new medical interventions and wellness products significantly impacts microbial populations. For example, excess fluoride can cause tooth discoloration and pitting, and some toothpaste abrasives can erode enamel.[82] Some sunscreen ingredients may disrupt hormones and harm marine life, and extensive use can reduce vitamin D production.[83] We also now know that antibiotics can selectively kill or inhibit the growth of certain bacteria. Certain medications are beneficial and harmful to many microbial species.

But killing all our microbes is not good. By now you see, we need them to live long and be healthy.

Harmonious Microbes, Vital You

Homeostasis is when the body is able to self-regulate and maintain stability while adjusting to conditions that are best for its survival.[84] In other words, we need our microbial communities to work harmoniously together. Remember this:

Homeostasis = Health

If we understand what microbes are doing to cause disease, we can take preventative measures and avoid molecular and cellular damage that leads to decline.

So, then, how do we keep them in balance? Ultimately, we need to be aware of the environments we expose our bodies to and their effects on our microbial communities. Equally important is our diet. Our ability to manage stress and engage in physical activity also plays a significant role. Moreover, our mindset is critically important, given the connection between our body and brain.

However, in addition to understanding these insights, there is a lot of trending advice on what to eat, how to lose weight, and how to look good. Should we go gluten-free? What about eating paleo or keto? Is plant-based eating better? Some people believe exercise is far more important than diet. Each person has their own "health religion." So, what actions should we take? What choices do we need to make?

Well, that's where we went to work, and what we'll dive into next is sharing our journey to find solutions.

The Mindset Shift

If you take one insight from this chapter, let it be this...

Staying healthy is about keeping your internal ecosystem in balance.

Health = Homeostasis.

Ultimately, to do this, you need to keep your microbes harmoniously working together.

Key Insights

- The Airbus A380 is a double-decker plane and one of the most complex machines. Miraculously, it has never crashed because engineers use an approach of continuous monitoring and maintenance. Once a part shows signs of wearing, it is immediately replaced. Viome uses a similar model for the human body.
- Our focus to digitize the human body drew our attention to the emerging field of microbiome science.
- The human body has about 40 trillion microbes.
- The activity of our microbes is fundamental for longevity and disease-free living.
- The microbiome has been linked to almost all diseases, from acute conditions—digestive issues, skin conditions, brain fog, headache, and mood—

to chronic diseases—immune conditions, heart disease, cancer, and neurological conditions.

- Superagers appear to have more microbial species in their microbiomes.
- The rise in disease rates is in great part a result of our modern lifestyles, which also cause our environments and food to be less microbially diverse than they once were.
- Additionally, positive modern health innovations like antibiotics and C-Sections have played a role in microbiome changes that have led to more disease.
- Homeostasis = Health. Achieving great health is about the body's ability to maintain homeostasis or stay in balance.

CHAPTER 4

INNOVATING IN THE ERA OF PRECISION MEDICINE

The biggest innovations of the 21st century will be at the intersection of biology and technology. A new era is beginning.

—*Steve Jobs*

My dad was not an entrepreneur. He was an engineer who worked for the government and thought business was risky. He always told me to "get a damn degree in accounting." He wanted me to have a secure, well-paying job. If I secured a stable 9-5 job with benefits, he would view it as a success. He experienced tremendous financial struggles in his early life, but that changed after signing his government employment contract. So, in his mind, that should have been the path forward for me.

On the other hand, my mom has always had this unshakable belief in me. So, whenever my dad launched his typical sermon, she'd shush him. She'd say, "Narendra, our boy is very intelligent. He can do whatever he wishes."

My mother taught me the sky's the limit. And I decided early on to believe her, which has benefited me greatly.

Out of purely good intentions, and often to protect us, there will always be people who create limits and urge us to be mindful of them. We live in a world where people try to contain us. Inadvertently, we may do it to others too. There are people like my dear old dad, who lovingly told me my best bet was to get a government job and stay with it until retirement. For him, doing anything else was wrong. But he was speaking from his belief system, worldview, and perspective on life. Over the years, as he watched me navigate life as an entrepreneur, he learned success was possible, and there was a formula to it.

Beliefs are merely choices that become self-fulfilling prophecies that hold us back. If you believe you can't because you're poor, a woman, or have brown skin, or you're too old, or money isn't for you, your behaviors will follow. You will reinforce your own limiting beliefs. So, remember that while people will try to contain you, your destiny is up to you.

My mom's "sky's the limit" mantra might explain why my best memories of my childhood are from my time spent stargazing. Many evenings, I would sit on a tree stump or a rock and look up at the inky black sky filled with twinkling pinpricks of light. I'd imagine that those tiny yet magnificent stars were the same ones that the richest person in the world was gazing at. And I realized our access to the starry sky was the same. We had the same view! And in those moments, I became the richest person in the world because I had the same power. I also realized I had a better view sitting in pitch-black darkness. The richest person in the world would be watching the sky from a fancy room in a city penthouse, wouldn't they? You can't even see the stars if hundreds of brightly lit skyscrapers surround you.

Early on, I learned that limitations were created. They were just ill-conceived artifacts of my restless monkey mind. I understood that what I believe is up to me, and I have the same ability as the most powerful people in the world. I learned that what we perceive as power is only pseudo-power. No one is better than anyone else. If you have a mind that is imaginative and an abundant, healthy body, there is nothing you can't achieve.

When my three children, Ankur, Priyanka, and Neil, were growing up, I always told them what my mom had told me. But then, in my thirties, I learned my mom was wrong, too. And then, my understanding of the world expanded beyond the sky because I realized the sky doesn't exist.

"The sky's the limit" was my mom's limitation. The sky is simply a figment of our imagination. When you **The truth is *we create our sky*.** go from here to the Moon, you don't pass the sky. There is no sky. You simply go from an experience of gravity to one of no gravity, and there is no "sky," and it goes on and on and on. You realize the Universe is one giant place with gravitational and non-gravitational elements.

The truth is *we create our sky*.

We create imaginary boundaries for ourselves when we buy into falsehoods like *I'm too old to do anything about my body*. Everyone creates their own sky. So, why not choose the empowering, abundant beliefs? After all, they require the same mental effort.

I tell you this because you must understand that innovation requires a limitless mind. And it is important to address that now, because it's what we will delve into next. You will shortly discover the personalized health innovations we developed at Viome. These solutions emerged from connecting the dots between the current scientific understanding of aging and disease and technology.

To innovate, I have learned, you must always remember there is no sky. You must be obsessed with solving the problem you set out to solve. I always tell entrepreneurs that you must have an obsession if you want to succeed at a moonshot.

Obsession is an almost maniacal force within you that propels you beyond your fears. In that state, you are driven so intensely that you want to learn every facet of the problem you are trying to solve. Then, the answers that emerge are crucial for creating a solution.

Passion does not have the same kind of power. It is a much weaker force. It is fine for hobbies like cooking, painting dog portraits, or learning yoga (unless, for you, those are obsessions!).

If you truly want to experience fulfillment and innovation, be obsessed with solving a problem. Whenever you hit an imaginary sky, remind yourself that it doesn't exist and keep going. If you're not obsessed, you will lose your way whenever you encounter an obstacle and simply stop to find a new passion.

The other remarkable thing about obsession is like attracts like. When you're obsessed, the people you need find you. They are drawn to you because you're a magnet. You become a nexus for the same problem they are passionate about. And this is when the real magic begins.

As our team grew, all the pieces began to fall into place. Each team member, like me, was obsessed with solving the problem of aging and illness, but from a different lens of expertise and life experience. Some taught me about the complexities of creating solutions for the human body, a system of systems full of microbes that determine health. Others were technologists who taught me how critical technologies like AI can be used for solving the world's greatest problems. I also had team members who understood the diet fad crazes and how they cause so many to struggle with weight and food.

Together our focus differed from that of other companies that offer treatments to manage symptoms. Our mission was to build a business that offers solutions that keep people healthy.

From the outset, I had to remind myself numerous times that limits are only in the mind. To be an innovator, you have to be okay with not knowing how it's going to go. You don't need all the answers. The key is to start with a moonshot that defines what you want to see happen in the future. Then, you evaluate the starting point. Next, you determine the first problem you need to solve to get closer to the end goal, and you start to work on that. Once you solve it, a new problem will surface, and then you select that as the next mission that will get you closer to the solution. And it goes like that.

So, when we launched Viome with the moonshot to make aging and illness optional, the first step was to get a group of expert minds together. This would enable us to build a biological intelligence platform, which was needed to process massive amounts of data that, when analyzed, would lead us to our first solutions. And so, our first mission in our moonshot was to create it. We called it Vie.

Mission #1: The quest for superior personalized health metrics.

The Goal: Give people personalized information and deeper insights about the state of their health by looking at microbial activity in their body so that they can take action to improve.

The Challenge: No one had successfully processed the level of biological data with an AI system that was truly needed to provide actionable health data. To do that, we needed a platform to analyze the data we collected from biological samples that people sent to our lab. We needed this to give them insights about what was happening in their bodies.

Our Solution: We built Vie, the world's most advanced biological intelligence platform.

Building the Most Advanced Biological Platform

Our first step was to build a biological intelligence platform. We knew this would require processing massive datasets and using AI was the solution. We began with the equation below (introduced in Chapter 3).

$$\text{Biological Intelligence} + \text{Human Intelligence} \times \text{Artificial Intelligence} = \text{Precision Health}$$

I knew that if we could combine these three elements in the right way, it would be the basis for Vie and the basis for our success as a company.

Now not only was Vie our first innovation, but it is behind every personalized health solution we've been able to create and bring to the world. So, let me explain how each element of the formula came into play and how the vision took shape. Let's start with Biological Intelligence.

Biological Intelligence

Biological Intelligence is the science of the human body. It is everything that scientists have learned since humans started investigating how the human body works thousands of years ago. It encompasses knowledge we have gathered along the way through to the present day. It includes what Hippocrates documented about 2400 years ago and is inclusive of breakthroughs in laboratories that are publishing results today.

We know, for instance, that the human body has an intrinsic tendency to self-organize. Just think how miraculous it is to be human. **The human body has an intrinsic tendency to self-organize.** We're born with this bio-container (our body), which allows us to get around and live our lives. It's one of the most complex systems in the world.

Our cells inherently know how to transform into the tissues and organs the body needs to function. The human body also has remarkable mechanisms built into it for prevention and repair. That's why when you cut your finger, your body grows new cells to fix blood vessels, skin, and other tissues to repair the wound. Our brains are also miraculous. Every day, we have approximately 70,000 thoughts using 100 billion neurons that connect at more than 500 trillion points.[85]

The human body has an aptitude for intelligence we still don't fully understand. However, we do know that everything is connected. The biology of the human body is a dynamic interplay between complex cellular, molecular, organ, and tissue systems, all of which can be impacted by the different nutrients and toxins that can come not only from our diet but can also be produced by all the trillions of microbes that live in us, from the oral cavity to the gut. By understanding what is happening in our bodies at the molecular level, we can understand why we get sick and what it takes to be healthy.

At Viome, our focus is on epigenetics, the study of how environmental influences affect gene activity. This expanding area of research reveals how aspects such as diet, nutrition, exercise, sleep, and our relationships impact our health. It's important to understand that gene expression controls the behavior of both microbial and human cells, which adapt continuously to changes in their environment.[86]

We use a specific epigenetic technology known as metatranscriptomics. This method involves analyzing RNA transcripts—copies of RNA used to synthesize proteins—created by the microbiome in a given environment. By examining these RNA molecules, we can identify which genes are being actively expressed at any moment. This analysis helps us understand the activities of microbes, indicating which genes might be expressed based on their actions.[87]

You may be familiar with the term epigenetics because it is a growing discipline. Recent discoveries have also led to breakthrough advances, such as mRNA

Vaccines, the groundbreaking vaccine technology used to treat COVID-19. The success of these vaccines has further led to the exploration of mRNA technology in other diseases, including cancer.[88]

The important point about epigenetics is that it focuses on RNA and tells us what is happening at the molecular level. It's different from static genetic tests, like those used for DNA interpretation.

Now, Biological Intelligence on its own is simply information. How we apply the information in the quest for a solution requires humans, which brings us to the second variable in the equation: Human Intelligence.

Human Intelligence

The variable Human Intelligence is the sum of collective wisdom (knowledge from current science) filtered by a team of expert thinkers.

I knew from experience that our mission would require a team of brilliant minds, and I needed to find them. That's why my first action was to share my moonshot with the world in the media. I knew that others who were obsessed with my mission would find me. And they did. Each new team member helped me understand new aspects of the problem, and that allowed us to start to formulate what we needed to get to the solutions.

People came to the team united by the mission, but each came with their own reason. You already know mine. At 57, I wanted to be like my superager great-grandmother and my Dadi and dodge the cancer that was my father's fate. My motivation for making illness optional was to avoid it myself and keep living my life to the fullest.

You know Momo's reason. He had an illness doctors couldn't solve and was compelled to build new solutions to solve major illnesses.

Guru, our CTO, had been personally affected by chronic illness too. But for him, it was his daughter who was fighting for her health. She suffered from a cluster of symptoms ranging from fatigue, allergies, flu-like symptoms, food sensitivities, and migraines during her high school years. Like Momo, Guru's daughter got an "idiopathic" diagnosis, which means no one expert fully understood what was wrong. So, Guru became committed to building new solutions to treat chronic illness, but from his lens of expertise, which is AI.

Another of the earliest calls I got was from Dr. Helen Messier. She has a Ph.D. in microbiology and her MD in functional medicine, a type of healthcare that focuses on understanding the underlying root cause of diseases. At the time, she was working for longevity pioneer Craig Venter. Her focus was to increase people's lifespans, but she thought, *What's the point of living longer if people are going to be sick anyway?* So, she left her job and joined us to focus on eradicating disease and helping people optimize their health.

Two other team members came next, and they helped me understand the challenges in the existing health and wellness markets. One was Dr. Stephen Barrie, our Head of Clinical Nutrition, who has taught me a great deal about the shortcomings in the current medical system.

Stephen has an obsession with helping physicians get to the root of health problems and improve the Western medical system. Like Dr. Messier, he is one of the world's top medical doctors in functional medicine. In the 1980s, he was working as a physician and realized that laboratory testing wasn't giving doctors the data they needed to treat diseases properly. Lab tests tell a medical professional how sick you are but not why you're sick. So, he formed a company called Genova Diagnostics, which became the world's largest functional medicine clinic. His obsession took him to China, where he worked with leaders in the field for nine years. He came to us shortly after that.

The other was my colleague Helene Vollbracht, our Head of Product Strategy and Brand. She taught me about the challenges for people, particularly women, navigating the wellness industry. Her story will be familiar to many women. Helene, working for another tech company, heard me being interviewed on a podcast and was compelled to join our mission, which aligned greatly with her interest in health. The interviewer was a thought leader who promoted the keto diet, which Helene followed then. She was blown away when she heard me discussing the power of the human microbiome and Viome's potential to change lives.

Helene was eating keto, which had major negative effects on her body. She had already tried many other diet fads, like fasting and eating high-protein. She was in the entertainment industry, an industry where looking good was a priority. Consequently, Helene drove herself crazy, trying to change her body without a basic understanding of biology. Like so many, she was looking for answers outside of herself, always thinking, *the less I eat, the better I'll look.*

At one point, she was only eating popcorn because she didn't know what to eat that wouldn't make her gain weight. Fad diets took a toll on her body and her health. She did not yet understand the magic of eating for her biology and healing her microbiome. When you give your body what it needs, it begins to function properly. Now, she's obsessed with showing people that to achieve your health and body goals, you don't have to have a painful, complicated relationship with food.

As you can see, each team member is obsessed with solving the problem of aging and illness, but from very different perspectives. Over the years, I have continued to learn from more of the experts who have joined us, along with the millions of people we serve. Their wisdom and different perspectives, combined with the fast-accelerating science of the microbiome, gave us one variable we needed in our success equation.

With the team assembled, I now had the necessary experts from critical specialties to consolidate the right knowledge needed to pursue our moonshot. Viome continues to leverage the latest peer-reviewed papers and breakthroughs, constantly learning from the incredible wealth of knowledge available to transform it into actionable insights for our users. Our approach not only brings these scientific advancements to life but also contributes back to the scientific community. We share our discoveries, allowing us to add to the collective understanding of health and wellness. This synergistic cycle of learning and contributing ensures that we remain at the forefront of innovation, delivering unparalleled benefits to our users.

Now, even though my team includes some of the smartest experts on the planet, processing that amount of data required a technological miracle. It's good that AI was at a stage where it could be used for that purpose and was readily available for us to put to the task.

It can take decades for scientific breakthroughs to happen and become mainstream knowledge and for solutions to be made available. This is where AI has been a major catalyst. And in our formula, notice that the first two variables are added together where the third (AI) is a multiplier.

Artificial Intelligence

The human body conveys information on a massive scale. By one estimate, it generates about 780 terabytes of data each year.[89] To help visualize that, think of each piece of data as a grain of sand and then imagine all the grains of sand on a tropical island beach. Just a square foot of beach can hold one million grains of sand.[90]

> The human body conveys information on a massive scale. By one estimate, it generates about 780 terabytes of data each year.

With that quantity of data to sift through, we need AI support to uncover patterns and understand the complexity of each individual's biology. It's why we knew we would need an AI engine to decipher a person's unique bioprint to give them invaluable data about their body. This would be required to ensure they knew how to keep their system balanced.

Our AI genius, Guru, and his team built algorithms and guidelines for Vie, so she understands how to interpret a mass of biological data points. And the magic of AI is that it gets better over time. With every sample Vie interprets, we learn about more patterns and connections that we contribute to the growing body of knowledge in precision medicine.

These three elements— Biological Intelligence (the science of the human body), Human Intelligence (the team), and Artificial Intelligence (the technology to process the data)—were how we created Vie, which was our first major step.

Now, at the time, most microbiome companies were also focused on identifying which microbes were present, whether they were dead or alive, without considering whether their activity was beneficial or harmful. Our focus, however, was on analyzing the activity of living microbes within each individual to understand how they impact a person's health.

To illustrate the difference, imagine a library filled with books where the books represent microbes. Most companies were merely cataloging the titles and authors without delving into the content of the books. They could tell you what books were on the shelves (what microbes were in your body) but not what stories they told or how those stories might influence a reader. In contrast, Viome's approach was akin to reading each book, understanding its plot, characters, and the impact it could have on the reader's mind and emotions. Moreover, we consider how each book affects different readers in unique ways based on their individual behaviors and histories.

Understanding what microbes are actively doing inside you and whether their activity is beneficial or harmful is crucial for combating aging and disease. Once you can measure and comprehend this information, you can take proactive measures. This knowledge informs what foods to eat to obtain the nutrients that improve microbial activity. Ultimately, when your microbes are optimized, so is your health.

Our goal was to provide actionable insights that people can use to know what to do to stay healthy. And so, once we had our platform, we still needed to populate it with data. We knew this would come from biological samples collected from our customers. But what samples should we target, and how would we collect them?

The answer was poop. Said another way, we looked at the gut.

Mission #2: Develop solutions that allow people to be in control of their health.

The Goal: Build personalized health tests that allow people to understand what is going on in their body and what to do to stay youthful and healthy.

The Challenge: Overcoming the need to see or wait for medical professionals or the healthcare system to improve to take control of a person's health. Until now, people have had to rely on the medical system, regulatory bodies, and the government to manage their health. Often, a patient would be sidelined while they waited for a solution and they would have little say in the process.

Our Solution: A suite of personalized at-home test kits with dynamic, actionable data that can be used to improve health.

Breaking Ground in Precision Health

Our scientists started with the most microbe-populated and accessible region in the body—the gut or digestive tract, which is the long tube running from the mouth through the torso to the bottom (or butt).

> Gut health is a key indicator of overall physical and mental well-being.

Gut health is a key indicator of overall physical and mental well-being. As Hippocrates, the father of

Western medicine, once said: "All diseases begin in the gut," and today, we have science that supports this early wisdom. The gut's primary role in the body is digestion, yet its importance extends far beyond that because it is connected to almost every other region of the body. Even your brain!

Besides digestion mechanisms, the gut contains billions of neurons, and they are no different from the ones in our heads. In fact, the gut produces 95 percent of the body's serotonin, a key neurotransmitter associated with good mood. It connects to the brain through a communication channel known as the gut-brain axis or vagus nerve.[91]

Have you ever had butterflies when you were excited or anxious? That's your gut-brain connection in action. As I mentioned in Chapter 3, we shouldn't think of the vagus nerve like the other famous Vegas we know—Las Vegas. It's the opposite. *What happens in the gut doesn't stay there. It goes everywhere!* Gut imbalance is the start of most diseases.

Here's one other mind-boggling fact about the gut: The gut is home to the enteric nervous system. Due to its size and complexity, it operates independently and in conjunction with the central nervous system. Our brains contain about 100 trillion neurons, while the gut has 600 million smart, tiny cells. To give you an idea of how sophisticated the gut is, think about the intelligence level of a small animal, like a dog or a cat. Spot and Fluffy are on the same level neuron-wise as the human gut. A dog has about 530 million neurons, while a cat has about 250 million.[92]

Evolutionary biologists say we have a brain in our gut to help our bodies be more efficient. It is similar to how a computer sends processes to the cloud. Our brains offload some functions by sending them to the gut, which makes us more efficient. [93]

The gut is also the body's epicenter of microbial activity.[94] Simply put, if the human body were the world, the gut would be China, the world's most populous country as of 2020. In fact, the number of microbes in our gut equals the combined human population of Earth (8 billion or so) times 5000.[95]

Its high microbial density made it the first area of focus when scientists started learning about the human microbiome. It is also an easily accessible body region, so collecting samples from the gut is relatively simple. With a small scoop of our poop (scientists call it a "fecal" or "stool" sample), we can gain invaluable information about your overall health. And we can do it without any invasive procedures. There are around 100 billion bacteria per gram of wet poop![96]

So, with this understanding of the gut microbiome, its connection to health, and Vie as our tool, our team came together to figure out how to build a solution. With data from gut samples, the question became how to use it to provide back preventive measures people could take to stay healthy. We started with one powerful lever of health that we all do everyday—eat!— and how to use food as medicine to avoid aging decline and disease.

Food is Medicine

For decades, we've been told to eat certain foods and avoid others. But our first and most critical breakthrough at Viome was the discovery that there are no universal foods that are good for all.

Data shows that what works for one person doesn't work for another. We call this *biochemical individuality*.

Our bodies need different foods at different times to stay healthy because each person has an individualized microbial makeup. In fact, even identical twins with the same DNA respond to the same food very differently.[97] So, broad-sweeping diet recommendations that assume that we're all the same are no longer valid. However, unfortunately there are many misconceptions around what is considered "good" food or "bad" food. This is one reason why obesity and chronic disease rates continue to soar.

It's not just the food we eat but what our microbiome does with that food that determines the status of our health. Sometimes, we eat foods that are seemingly healthy, but if our microbes are unable to digest these foods or are converting them into harmful substances, then so-called "healthy" foods can be harmful.

Since all foods are made of chemicals that react with the chemicals in our bodies, depending on the mix, this can lead to good or bad health effects. So, to stay vital, you need to understand data obtained from your body and use chemistry and math to calculate accurate and personalized food and diet recommendations. Your biology should inform you exactly what you need to do.

If you are struggling with this new way to eat, think about it this way: If we present the same symptoms to three different nutritionists, we will likely get three different nutritional recommendations. But this is not how the scientific method works. What would you think if you asked three mathematicians, "What is 2+2?" and you received three different answers? You would say they're crazy.

There is a new, more sophisticated way to eat to stay healthy, and it's called Precision Nutrition or Nutrition 2.0. It's eating what your body needs to stay in balance. With each sample we process, we continue to learn how the foods many people think are healthy contribute to negative symptoms.

Let's digest all this with some real-life examples so you see how eating—something we all do every day—is critical for staying healthy. And how it's very important to know what foods to eat and when.

As I mentioned earlier in this book, a common food people think is healthy is spinach. There are people who think it's the ultimate superfood. Popeye taught us that if we eat it, it will make us strong because it contains iron and has vitamins like folate and fiber in it. But, as you now know, it's also one of the highest sources of oxalates. When oxalates bind to certain minerals, like calcium, magnesium, and iron, they prevent us from absorbing them, which impacts our health. Our gut microbes metabolize oxalates in the diet. However, some people's gut microbiomes don't have this ability. They can lead to issues like kidney stones.[98]

Another food with a great reputation is grapefruit. It's often thought of as a superfood for weight loss. It's low in calories and high in water and fiber. However, a compound in grapefruit blocks the enzyme that breaks down cortisol in the body. Cortisol is our stress hormone. It contributes to cravings and weight gain. With grapefruit blocking this enzyme, cortisol stays elevated.[99] So, for someone who struggles with elevated cortisol, avoiding grapefruit may enable them to lose weight.

Turmeric is also often praised for its anti-inflammatory benefits. However, it can cause inflammation by stimulating the production of bile acids released by the gallbladder into our intestines to help us digest fats in the diet. When the gut microbiome is unbalanced, microbes can metabolize that bile acid and send it back to the liver rather than getting rid of it. It can also lead to inflammation and fatty liver.[100]

Broccoli is another good guy/bad guy. It is touted for its anti-cancer benefits, and rightfully so. However, the same beneficial sulfur compounds can be harmful. Microbes in the gut use sulfur compounds and foods like broccoli to produce sulfide gas, which leads to digestive upset, gas, bloating, and inflammation in the gut.[101]

While coffee may be a cornerstone of many people's morning routine, it may not be ideal for everyone. Coffee offers several benefits with its polyphenol content. For some people, it helps increase cellular energy production by activating the genes involved in the mitochondria.[102]

However, caffeine may cause harm to other people by increasing stress hormones that negatively impact the gut microbiome and digestive motility. It can lead to issues like constipation or diarrhea.

So, anytime you hear that a food or supplement is good for everyone, you shouldn't eat it unless your name happens to be "Everyone." I'm kidding, of course, but please understand that there is no such thing as a universal healthy food or supplement. Roman philosopher Titus Lucretius Carus (known simply as Lucretius) coined the expression in the first century BC: "quod ali cibus est aliis fuat acre venenum" which means: "what is food for one man may be bitter poison to others." In other words, one man's food is another man's poison.

At the outset of our journey, we knew we didn't just want to give people information without also providing recommended actions. Many tests on the market just provide a simple static picture of a person's health. So, it was always our goal to offer solutions that would show people how their health is trending and what they can do to improve it, no matter where they're starting. And so, processing stool samples early in our journey gave us the first insights we needed to begin to connect unhealthy microbial activity to food so we could offer preventive measures.

Ultimately, this thinking and work led to our first affordable at-home precision health solution, a test kit we still offer today called the Gut Intelligence Test™.

Balanced Gut, Vital You

The development of our Gut Intelligence Test integrates microbiome science, AI, and stool sample collection to create preventive solutions via an at-home test. Using this test, anyone can collect a pea-sized stool sample at home and send it to our lab. Once we receive it, we analyze the stool and then provide personalized reports based on the data we collect.

When designing our first at-home test, we faced the challenge of adapting scientific health tests typically used by trained medical professionals. Our aim was to create a test that anyone could use at home that would provide understandable, actionable, and useful results. We now can translate billions of data points from the gut into twenty gut health scores. These are the foundation of the recommendations we send back to the user via our platform and mobile app.

Our sequencing technology allows us to understand inflammatory activity, if a person is having trouble breaking down certain foods and if the gut is properly absorbing nutrients. We can also determine if microbes are producing the molecules that are causing problems or are beneficial. We can even gain insights into microbes impacting blood sugar response. And all this is done in a short time. The analysis typically takes 10-12 days, from when the lab receives a sample to when scores are shared back. Users receive scores with preventative or correctional measures they should take to achieve internal balance.

We provide two types: 1) functional and 2) pathway activity scores. And while we could write an entire book on each, we've kept it to a high level for this book. To learn more, visit TheYouthFormula.com.

To help our customers use food as medicine, we categorize food items into four groups: Avoid, Minimize, Enjoy, and Superfood. We explain which foods are beneficial or harmful for you, provide the reasoning, and specify how long to avoid certain foods. Each recommendation is based on your body's data and designed to address critical areas of health:

- ✓ Enhance nutrient uptake for maximum nutrient absorption.
- ✓ Stimulate beneficial gut microbes to increase butyrate production.
- ✓ Inhibit the activity of harmful gut bacteria and reduce the risk of toxic byproducts like LPS, TMA, gas, and uremic toxins.
- ✓ Reinforce the gut lining to minimize the risk of "leaky gut" and improve digestive health.
- ✓ Address the underlying factors contributing to chronic inflammation.
- ✓ Personalize your dietary approach to optimize blood sugar levels and minimize food-related symptoms.

✓ Slow biological aging by addressing activities contributing to oxidative stress and inflammation throughout your body.

Our customized food lists have information on over 300 foods. After a test is complete, we recommend eating and avoiding certain foods for 4–6 months. While a person may need to avoid a favorite food for that period of time, it doesn't mean they can't have it again. The microbiome is always changing, especially as diet changes are made. Therefore, the foods you need now may differ from those you need in six months. We suggest people retest every six months to measure progress.

It's been incredible to see patterns emerge from each sample we process. Precision nutrition continues to show major promise and I believe in the future we will all eat according to our biochemical individuality.

At Viome, we have tracked people who follow a plan for about two to four months to understand the impact of diet modification on conditions like IBS, depression, anxiety, and type two diabetes. Here are some incredible results we've published:

- People with severe IBS saw a 39 percent improvement, while those with mild to moderate cases saw a 50 percent improvement. The success rate of a precision diet is about the same as that of most IBS medications, without any side effects.
- In depression and anxiety, our research showed a 31 percent improvement in severe cases. Compared to antidepressants, this is promising. It showed that diet is effective about 20 to 30 percent of the time.

- For type 2 diabetes, we saw a 30 percent reduction in relative risk.

To read more on our peer-reviewed studies and results, visit Viome.com/publications.

We can ultimately eat our way into disease, but we can also eat our way out of it. Hippocrates wisely said, "Let food be thy medicine," and when it comes to gut health, this couldn't be more true. Every sample we process reinforces this idea.

Still, once we started providing targeted food recommendations (from testing stool samples), we realized we could access more accurate data and provide deeper, better insights if we added two more sample types that would be simple to collect using an at-home test kit: 1) saliva and 2) blood.

We included saliva analysis because the mouth, like the gut, is easily accessible, and it is the body's second most densely populated microbiome region. The mouth is also the starting point for many diseases and is closely linked to overall health.

Then, we added a blood test because cellular health, in addition to microbial health, provides the most robust picture of overall health. These additions led to our second innovation and precision health solution, the Full Body Intelligence Test™.

Full Body Health—Going Beyond the Gut

Most of us diligently brush our teeth every morning and each night in pursuit of fresh breath, a healthy smile, and pearly white teeth. No one wants to look like Jack Sparrow. Yet, good oral health is important beyond mere aesthetics. Most people don't realize that the mouth is the starting point for numerous systemic diseases.

Healthcare professionals have recognized for years that oral problems, such as periodontitis—a severe gum infection—can lead to chronic issues elsewhere in the body.[103] However, rarely does the average person pat themselves on the back after they brush and floss because their nightly routine has helped them avoid other major chronic conditions like type 2 diabetes, heart disease or cancer, or a long list of major cognitive conditions. But consider these findings:

- An astounding 95 percent of people with diabetes have periodontal disease, highlighting the mouth's critical connection to overall health.[104]
- Those with compromised oral health are more likely to develop Alzheimer's.[105]
- Individuals with poor oral health are at a greater risk of developing various forms of cancer, from lung and colorectal cancer to pancreatic and breast cancer.[106]

The correlations are startling and underscore the profound impact of oral health on full-body health.

Women with poor oral health may also face more adverse pregnancy outcomes, including preterm births and low birth rates.[107] Simply knowing this can be a wake-up call for any woman or couple reading this who is contemplating pregnancy. An oral health check should be a top priority for couples trying to conceive and preparing for a birth, followed by proactive measures to enhance oral well-being.

While a beautiful smile is a compelling reason for oral care, now you can see that research from the past few decades has revealed benefits that extend far beyond vanity. So, we incorporated saliva as an important part of our test solutions.

Next, we added a blood test because, without it, we were missing invaluable information on cellular activity. We realized if we were going to offer solutions in health and aging, we would need to understand the state of a person's cellular health too, because virtually every element of our makeup consists of cells. They are the basic building blocks of all living things, making up tissues, organs, and, ultimately, the organ systems that allow our bodies to function. This would also give us invaluable insights into a cell's operation and how it lives, grows, and reproduces. We call that cellular health. [108]

After the addition of a blood sample, we were able to examine how well your cells handle stress and whether they need additional nutrient support. If oxidative stress shows up as an issue in your health, you may find antioxidant recommendations on your list of recommendations to help promote balance and neutrality in your cells. Your scores might also show supplements you need to take to help optimize how well your cells protect your DNA.

With the rollout of the Fully Body Intelligence Test, integrating analysis of stool, blood, and saliva allowed us to provide a detailed picture of health and offer back superior recommendations on preventative measures a person needs to stay healthy.

The test also includes a Biological Age measurement. It indicates how well or poorly your body is functioning relative to your actual age. It is a better predictor of health, risk of age-related diseases, and mortality than chronological age. Using it, I discovered that although I am chronologically 65 years old, my biological age is 52!

Our ability today to extract such detailed data was unimaginable a decade ago. With our Full Body Intelligence Test, we can now collect comprehensive phenotype data on individuals.

This data-driven approach provides the most comprehensive personalized nutrition advice and or disease prevention.

Once we got there, we realized that preventative food measures were a key component of what would keep people healthy but it wasn't enough. With the nutritional decline in today's food, our modern lifestyle, and a myriad of unproven wellness products on the market, we needed to do more. We had to figure out how to tackle these challenges with solutions that counteract how a multitude of problems of modern life lead to microbiome imbalance and disease. Our focus turned next to innovative preventative health measures.

Mission #3: Find a way for people to stay healthy even if the nutritional quality of our food remains a problem and our modern lifestyle puts pressure on our bodies.

The Goal: Create preventive health solutions that address the epidemic of declining nutritional quality in our food and ineffective, mass-market supplements, questionable wellness products, and modern life.

The Challenge: Our food is less nutritionally dense than it used to be due to soil depletion, modern farming techniques, harsh chemicals, and engineered foods. As a result, our bodies can no longer obtain the necessary nutrients from food alone to prevent disease and early aging. Additionally, industrialized living and the products we use are causing the extinction of beneficial microbes, which has negative health implications.

Today, we need supplements to stay healthy. However, most supplements offer generic solutions and lack sufficient education on what is best for individual needs. Additionally, we are not doing enough to prevent disease at its starting point—the mouth—before it reaches the gut.

Our Solution: Personalized health products designed for each individual's unique microbiome.

Leading the Charge on Preventive Health Measures

If you're like most people, you commonly visit the vitamin aisle at the pharmacy or grocery store, stare blankly at a wall of bottles, and select what you think you need because you heard about it from a family member or saw it on the web. *Superagers take Omega 3! NAD, the anti-aging miracle supplement! North Americans Need Vitamin D.* Being informed about supplements is important because it is easy to waste money or make choices that lead to negative health outcomes.

Think about it this way: If you tried to make a salad, but threw a bunch of confusing ingredients together— let's say, lettuce, anchovies, turmeric, and pickles . . . *bleh*—it would taste bad and be a waste of time. It might even be bad for your body. Yet, this is what most people do with supplements. People tend to think the higher the UI level on the bottle, the better. But do you even know what a UI is? It's a way of quantifying how much a vitamin should have an effect on your body.[109] So, a higher UI doesn't mean it's best for you. In fact, most dosage recommendations in supplement bottles are for healthy people. They don't consider what your body needs from an individual perspective.

Instead, when selecting supplements, we should ask the following questions: *Which specific nutrients is my body lacking? Why isn't my body making enough of them? Why does my body need these particular nutrients? When are they most crucial? What quantities should I consume for optimal health?*

Supplements play a crucial role in complementing our diets, especially as the nutritional value of modern foods has declined and our bodies face an onslaught of stressors.[110] Sometimes, we need to eat an item in large amounts to get the necessary nutrients. Other times, our gut microbiome may not agree with certain foods, even though they contain nutrients essential for our health.

For instance, one common supplement today is NAD, short for nicotinamide adenine dinucleotide. It has drawn attention for its purported anti-aging benefits. It's sought after for its potential to replenish declining NAD levels in our body as we age, with early research—primarily in mice and yeast—suggesting it could extend lifespan and improve mitochondrial health and muscle regeneration.

But, the body's response to supplements like NAD is highly individualized. While some may benefit from increased NAD levels, others must be cautious. Individuals with a high presence of senescent or zombie cells—cells that have stopped dividing and contribute to inflammation—might find that boosting NAD could inadvertently support the survival of these problematic cells, potentially worsening inflammation.[111] It's crucial to consider personal health markers and potential risks before deciding to supplement with NAD.

Acetyl L-carnitine is a natural substance in your body, foods, and supplements that can help improve your brain function and energy levels. However, people who produce a lot of a certain gut chemical called TMAO should be careful. This chemical is linked to poor heart health and an increased risk of heart disease. Taking acetyl L-carnitine can raise TMAO levels even more, which might increase the risk of heart problems.[112]

Also, if your body produces a lot of harmful toxins called uremic toxins, you should be cautious with tyrosine supplements. These toxins build up in the blood mainly when the kidneys aren't working well and can't get rid of them. Tyrosine can turn into substances that increase these toxins, making the problem worse.[113]

As it is with food, supplementation is personal. And so, we started to offer tailored recommendations.

Personalized Supplements

We now offer custom formulas for each individual, ensuring that everyone receives precisely what their body needs down to the milligram. We patented a mechanism that allows us to determine what foods and supplements a person needs based on the analysis of their gut microbiome, oral microbiome, and human gene expression. We also received a patent on producing made-to-order custom supplements that only include the ingredients that your body needs in only the dosage that your body needs.

Dosages of vitamins and minerals are determined based on efficacious research of the amounts used in clinical studies to help improve a certain condition. So, in some cases, the amounts may be higher than the percent daily value (%DV). Most people don't understand that the term "100% DV" is a term the U.S. government uses. It defines an amount just above what is needed to keep from developing a specific nutrient-deficiency disease, such as scurvy, which is caused by a vitamin C deficiency.[114]

Oftentimes, dosages higher than 100% DV are needed in order to improve pathway activity. Viome has implemented safety checks in the recommendation process to ensure dosages do not exceed tolerable upper limits also set by the US government. When considering how much you need of a particular ingredient, we consider the dosages used in clinical trials, the severity of suboptimal scores, and the stage of life. From our tests, we provide recommendations for:

- Vitamins
- Digestive enzymes
- Polyphenols
- Amino acids
- Minerals
- Herbs

We also provide personalized probiotic and prebiotic solutions essential for gut health. Personalized recommendations feature safe strains that promote gut health and avoid those that could have negative effects.

People often think that "personalized" means expensive. But we also found a way to use robotics and artificial intelligence to reduce costs. Robots don't care if they make the same supplement once or a million times. Once you build an automated system, it's the same cost, so we've kept supplements under the price of a cup of cappuccino per day.

I believe precision supplements will undoubtedly be the future, and this is where we've been a leader. And we've also recently taken our supplements a step further.

We are currently integrating information from other apps. For instance, if we see you are not sleeping well, we can increase the amount of magnesium you get to help you sleep better.

These initial preventative measures to counteract nutritional deficiency were a good place to start, but next, we thought about how to build a solution to avoid disease states long before they start. So we widened our investigation to include the mouth. Could we build solutions that would stop diseases at the outset where they can begin—in the mouth?

Bringing Balance to the Mouth

Personalized food recommendations are a critical part of oral hygiene, but we realized we had to go a step further and target oral health, so we developed personalized lozenges and pH-balancing toothpaste that we formulate using saliva test scores.

By collecting small saliva samples using a simple procedure that takes only minutes, we can gain insights into overall health. This test currently offers sixteen oral health scores, and it provides data that allows us to offer personalized food and biotic recommendations that, when followed, can address the microbial imbalance and inflammation in the mouth and body.

We can see microbes that increase or decrease the prevalence of cavities, activities that promote cavity production, and microbe activities that influence the local pH. We can also assess pro-inflammatory pathways that also degrade and damage the gums; pathways that are associated with gingivitis and periodontal disease.

Currently, no other company offers this level of insight into the oral microbiome. In our saliva evaluation, we also pay close attention to breath odor because it is greatly affected by microbes. Individuals suffering from halitosis (the medical term for bad breath) often feel they've tried every possible hygiene and dental care solution without success. To address this, we provide assessments that pinpoint the specific microbial activities causing the odor, thereby offering targeted solutions. Moreover, our analysis extends to other crucial factors, such as the activity of oral pathogens.[115]

We have learned how critical it is to have a balanced pH in the mouth for overall health and disease prevention. And so, our personalized oral lozenges and toothpaste introduce biotics and nutrients directly to the mouth and throat.

The lozenges and toothpastes contain ingredients that help create protective microbial communities and support important activities in the mouth. They reduce gum inflammation and decrease the presence of pathogens linked to periodontal disease and cavities. Additionally, these products include elements that have been clinically proven to reduce sore throats, pharyngitis, and ear infections while boosting the body's natural immune defenses. They are also crafted without any harmful substances.

I am proud to say these preventative health solutions have now become a part of so many people's nightly routines. They brush, floss, and carry out the usual oral hygiene practices, then finish by popping a mint lozenge in their mouth. It dissolves, and its components go to work.

Our work in saliva analysis and oral health also led to a miracle breakthrough that brought our scientific endeavor and innovation focus to the realm of early detection diagnostics and therapeutics. Viome now offers an at-home test to detect biomarkers associated with early-stage oral and throat cancer.

Mission #4: Early detection of major diseases.

The Goal: Develop a model to improve early diagnosis of disease.

The Challenge: Diseases are difficult to detect in the early stages, and the sooner we catch them, the more we can improve outcomes or stop them long before we experience the first symptoms. Big data systems have previously been a challenge. However, now by using AI to make sense of biological data, we can gain deeper insights and connect the dots to see patterns and develop systems to prevent diseases long before they start.

Our Solution: Oral cancer early disease detection technology.

Tackling Early Disease Detection

Imagine if we could detect life-threatening and debilitating chronic diseases, like cancer, diabetes, or Parkinson's, long before symptoms arise, at the earliest stage while they're still curable. We know that diseases don't appear overnight but over several years, if not decades. So, why not focus on prevention? Doesn't that make logical sense?

While it does, unfortunately, the design of our current healthcare system is to prioritize the treatment of disease over prevention and early detection. As I explained earlier in this book, this is because our current system was built at a different time before the rates of chronic disease ballooned into what they are today. There are numerous challenges when it comes to prioritizing prevention. First of all, prevention campaigns are expensive and even if they were initiated, it would take decades to see results. Also, as we have discussed, most healthcare companies today profit from treating disease, not preventing it.

It's why the current approach in healthcare is reactionary and not proactive. We see this with conventional lab tests, for instance. They measure what exists, not the degree of pathology or the markers that explain "why" it exists. It's a fundamental issue in healthcare. Our current system focuses on detection and getting ahead of early signals of disease, which eventually leads to serious illness. However, a focus on being proactive and catching diseases early is the only way to stop them from escalating into serious fatal conditions.

Today, the approach to categorizing diseases is also flawed. Many chronic diseases share common origins and root problems. For instance, low-grade inflammation and microbial imbalance are the starting points for most diseases, including diabetes, renal and kidney failure, and cognitive impairments like Alzheimer's. These same biological factors manifest as different diseases depending on the individual and the context.

Early detection and intervention are crucial for addressing root causes before they escalate into severe health problems. The early stages of disease often present subtle, non-specific symptoms that are easily overlooked. However, these early signals are critical opportunities for intervention. By identifying and addressing these initial disturbances, we can prevent minor symptoms from escalating into life-threatening conditions. For example, low-grade inflammation, if left unchecked, can progress into chronic inflammation, a known precursor to serious diseases such as cancer, cardiovascular disease, and autoimmune disorders.

Recognizing these challenges, Viome pioneered a new approach to oral healthcare. Unlike conventional methods that rely heavily on visual and tactile exams and often miss subtle, early indicators of disease, Viome's Oral Health Pro™ CancerDetect™ uncovers the intricate interplay between microbial activities and human gene expression. This approach not only enhances the accuracy of early disease detection but also provides deeper insights into the root causes of oral and throat cancers.

Oral Health Pro detects early biomarkers associated with oral and throat cancer, such as bad breath, fungal activity, genotoxic activity, and more. With a specificity of 95 percent and sensitivity of 90 percent,[116] as documented in the Oral Oncology Journal, this test is the most advanced oral and throat cancer screening tool available today.

In the future, our groundbreaking technology will enable us to continue to develop new life-saving tests for early-stage cancers and many other life-threatening conditions. By leveraging predictive models, it is our aim to offer unprecedented precision in early detection and intervention and pave the way for a healthier future where proactive care significantly improves outcomes.

Also on the horizon for us is the possibility of developing customized therapeutics. Similar to food and supplements, our bodies respond to vaccines and drugs differently. That means early detection of disease and may include personalized drugs that make treatment more effective and help us avoid side effects.

Another major focus is to deepen our understanding of additional factors affecting microbiome health, including stress, physical activity, and sleep patterns. We're excited about what simple lifestyle tweaks can do to enhance well-being and extend lifespan.

As we advance in our scientific knowledge, we anticipate discovering more personalized health innovations. The pursuit of science and innovation is endless. And as long as people are sick and aging, we plan to keep pursuing our moonshot.

Frontiers for Future Discovery

For the entrepreneurs out there, remember this: Innovation thrives on insights obtained from new sources of data and scientific breakthroughs. Capturing better data helps you identify patterns and ultimately assists in designing new solutions. Data enables us to create life-saving tests and continually improve our products and services. You win in business and life when each version you create is more sophisticated than the last.

Mission-driven companies, rather than those solely focused on profit, thrive on learning, innovation, and technological advancements. It takes a different mindset to run a business that succeeds without exploitation and is not overly focused on profits. But this is how you become an innovator who carves a unique path in an industry.

Our work has made us a leader in the precision health space. Although there are other businesses in the field, most focus on DNA analysis, not RNA. They also emphasize symptom treatment rather than prevention or optimization. There is no doubt in my mind that, in the near future, and with the current attention surrounding the microbiome generating interest from more consumers, there will be more innovators entering our space.

Our next focus will be to explore the microbiomes of the skin and respiratory tract, and we may also progress to the microbiomes of genital regions. However, there is already a strong innovator in that latter segment called Evvy. It's a company I have full confidence in recommending because it was created and is owned by my daughter Priyanka Jain.

Evvy is a women's health company that offers vaginal health test kits. Since vaginal discomfort is one of the main reasons women seek healthcare advice, and over 90 percent of these cases are due to imbalances in the vaginal microbiome, Evvy's mission is to identify and use overlooked female biomarkers, starting with the vaginal microbiome. An imbalance can manifest as yeast infections, bacterial vaginosis (BV), cytolytic vaginosis (CV), aerobic vaginitis (AV), and more.[117]

I am tremendously proud of Priyanka for bringing health equality to women worldwide. She was the one who told me that until 1993 women weren't used as participants in medical research and drug development! When she told me this, I was shocked. Most of the drugs we take today have never been tested on women. It is almost unfathomable since we all come from a woman, and half of the population on the planet is female. Optimal health also starts at birth when babies transit their mom's birth canal.

I am even more proud because she once said she hated science and technology. And I tell you this story because it may inspire other women to consider careers in STEM fields, and if you are a parent, it might give you a chuckle too.

Many years ago, she came to me and said, "Dad, I know you love science and technology, but I have no interest." Apparently, at sixteen, she had found her passion.

At this point, many dads would say, *Sweetie, whatever your passion is, I'll help you get there!* But that's not what this dad did. I told her that she was too young to know her passion. I realized I hadn't done my job to expose her to the various possibilities in the world. So, I made a deal with her. If she went to Singularity University for four weeks to learn about nanotechnology, neuroscience, genetics, and artificial intelligence and then came to the same conclusion, I would support her. She rolled her eyes, but she went.

Four weeks later, she came to me sheepishly but with a twinkle in her eye. She told me she had decided to become a neuroscientist or a geneticist. When I asked her what changed her mind, she explained that in high school, all they did in science class was mix solutions and make colored liquid. She didn't see how there was any relevance to what they were doing in connection to the real world. Spending time with scientists and technologists taught her how science and technology are powerful tools for her to do what she wanted to do, which was to help girls and women succeed. And now that is what she does with Evvy.

Priyanka attended Stanford University and became both a Stanford STEM Fellow and a Stanford Mayfield Fellow. For those unfamiliar with the term STEM, it stands for Science, Technology, Engineering, and Mathematics. It's an educational approach that integrates these four disciplines into a cohesive learning model based on real-world applications. It's an approach that aims to equip students with critical thinking, problem-solving, and creative skills necessary to thrive in the 21st century's tech-driven world.

When Priyanka graduated, she joined a startup, her first company, which used AI to remove gender bias. Then, in 2021 when she learned about microbiome science, she launched Evvy, a women's health company that sells vaginal health test kits.

Evvy's test kits involve a swab to collect a sample from the vaginal microbiome. Any woman can do the test to understand if she has an imbalanced vaginal microbiome that may be causing infertility, pregnancy complications, or reveal sexually transmitted infections (STIs) and possibly even cancer.

So, if you're a woman seeking support, especially for those trying to get pregnant, know that Evvy is a solution you can tap into. To learn more, visit Evvy.com.

Great Health is Personal, and It's Complex

Given the intricacies of the human body, it's undeniable that systems biology is the only rational approach to healthcare. Unlike traditional methods that rely on reductionist (non-integrative) practices, systems biology considers the entire spectrum of life, integrating it into human health.

Our current healthcare system operates in silos, treating the body as separate parts. For kidney issues, you see a urologist; for heart problems, a cardiologist; for dental concerns, a dentist; for mental health, a psychiatrist. This fragmented approach fails to recognize the profound connections between mind and body and the multitude of factors affecting both.

This outdated model needs a complete overhaul. The future of healthcare lies in a systems-based approach, which is inherently holistic and acknowledges the incredible complexity of our bodies. The body's systems are more than just the sum of their parts—they interact in intricate and dynamic ways.

We must also remember that health is deeply personal. Each body is unique, requiring different things at different times. We now have the data to prove this individuality. Effective healthcare must consider five critical areas: nutrition, stress, fitness, sleep, and mindset.

Next, let's delve deeper into these five areas. I also have a simple formula for you that, with the knowledge you've gained in this book, makes it clear what steps to take for optimal health.

The Mindset Shift

If you take one insight from this chapter, let it be this...

The era of precision medicine is here, and it's growing. There was once a time when we didn't have the technology to see what was happening in our bodies. But today, we have those tools.

Viome has been an innovator. We're transforming health by creating tools that, for the first time, allow us to gain insights into what certain foods do to our bodies at a molecular level. We're also focused on prevention and being proactive.

We have learned that the new way to eat is a precision diet.
If you are eating foods without knowing if they are good for you, it's time to upgrade your approach.

Key Insights

- Obsession is needed for successful innovation. Passion is for hobbies.
- The formula Human Intelligence + Biological Intelligence x AI-Technology is about bringing the right experts together and looking at the problem through the right lens of science and technology. This formula was the basis for Vie, Viome's

AI platform and current suite of personal health solutions.

- Current solutions in health and wellness are focused on treating symptoms not getting to the root. Treatments and products are prescribed once a person is sick, not to prevent it from happening. Our current healthcare system is designed to profit from the sick.
- Viome is focused on ensuring people stay healthy.
- Our first solution was focused on gut health. The gut, also called the second brain, is the most densely populated microbiome in the human body.
- There are around 100 billion bacteria per gram of wet stool.
- Once we created our first innovation, The Gut Intelligence at-home kit, we learned how every person's body is different. Food is one way to restore the balance of the microbiome. However, with the nutritional value diminishing from food, personal supplementation became a focus.
- Viome is a leader in personalized supplements. By analyzing data from each person's individual microbiome, we engineer supplements to the mg that help bring balance to the body. Probiotics and prebiotics are part of our supplement solution.
- Since disease states begin in the mouth, we can stop many disease states even before they happen in the gut. We have innovated in oral health with mouth lozenges and toothpaste to balance mouth pH.
- Early detection and intervention are crucial for addressing root causes before they escalate into severe health problems.

- Viome has created the most advanced oral and throat cancer screening tool, Oral Health Pro with Cancer Detect, available today.
- As science continues to advance and we learn more we continue to explore other areas of the body and how factors such as exercise, sleep, and stress impact microbial communities in addition to food.
- For women, we recommend Evvy vaginal test kits.
- Great health is determined by many factors and how they impact the body. We need to think about the body as a system within systems. We also need to remember that our body is unique. Collecting data from our bodies helps us know what to do to stay healthy.

CHAPTER 5

BODY KNOWS BEST

*Healthy habits are learned in the same way as
unhealthy ones - through practice.*

—*Wayne Dyer*

What would have happened if the precision medicine
tools available today had been available twenty years
before my father died? Rarely do I ruminate about the
past, but I've had moments when I've had this thought.
Would I have been able to help my dad avoid his health
issues, both the aneurysm and prostate cancer, that
he survived? What about the pancreatic cancer that
took him from us? Could I have helped him avoid that
altogether and extended his life? I like to think that it
would have been possible.

Unfortunately, our breakthroughs at Viome in the last decade came too late for my dad. But I have been able to help my mom. Early on in this book, I told you she had high blood pressure and diabetes. After losing my dad, health became a greater focus, and she has made remarkable progress in the last few years.

One of the best things I've done in my life is to get my mom on Viome. The day she told me her doctor said she no longer needed an inhaler for her asthma, we celebrated. And not long after she got rid of the walker she once used. Now she is able to walk on her own. She told me, "Son, you have become a really good doctor."

Every six months, she calls me to say: "Naveen, where is my test kit?" She knows when it is time to test herself to the point where it's become a positive habit. She also takes precision supplements based on her test results. I am grateful to have the awareness, insights, and tools to help her access the new and evolving world of Nutrition 2.0 that's helping her and millions more achieve better health.

I have watched her make tremendous progress, and what I have learned over the last few years in our work is that measurement is the key. If you can measure a biomarker in the human body, then you can develop strategies to counteract or optimize it.

If you can measure a biomarker in the human body, then you can develop strategies to counteract or optimize it.

But, of course, ensuring balanced nutrition is only part of achieving optimal health. If you are working on your wellness, you know that there are other factors. Besides nutrition, they include stress management, sleep, and physical fitness. And there's a fifth one, purpose, that may not be immediately obvious but shows up in longevity studies as a key health indicator in superagers.

As health became a deep focus of mine, I noticed how much conflicting information exists in the health and wellness industries because of competing interests, personal bias, and money-making agendas. Knowing what to do to stay healthy can be difficult. So, to develop a better strategy, I began considering how to structure the vast scientific knowledge derived from years of research and data to make managing a person's health simpler.

As I considered these factors and how they are interrelated, I realized that we needed a framework to define them and keep them focused. I've also found there is a sequence to them, and that slightly new way to think about these five areas helps us consider what actions we need to take to stay healthy.

Lifestyle Over Genetics

As I thought about how to organize the five critical areas of health, I was inspired by a theory that has been around for decades that you've likely heard about: Maslow's Hierarchy of Needs.

It's a framework developed by American psychologist Abraham Maslow and published in 1943 that explains human motivation.[118]

Maslow's model, structured as a pyramid, suggests that humans are motivated by a series of hierarchical needs, starting with the most basic physiological necessities and ascending to the peak of self-actualization. He suggested that all people are motivated by five needs that he characterized in five categories: 1) physiological, 2) safety, 3) love and belonging, 4) esteem, and 5) self-actualization. The hierarchy suggests that humans must satisfy lower-level needs before pursuing higher-level psychological and self-fulfillment desires, influencing behavior and personal growth. He asserted that if one need is unmet, a person cannot advance up the hierarchy to achieve the next need.[119]

Figure 5.1—Maslow's Hierarchy of Needs

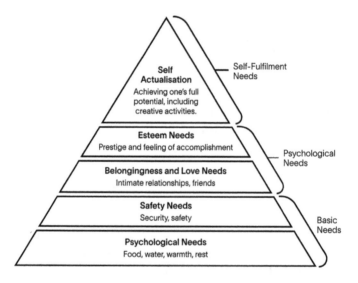

Maslow's Hierarchy of Needs simplifies and categorizes the complex array of human motivations into a structured model, visually represented as a pyramid.

While Maslow's approach was highly adopted when it was introduced and is still referenced today, it was never definitively proven. Still, it is a model that offers a clever approach. It's also used to this day because it's one of the best models to make aspects of the complexities of living understandable and actionable.

His model suggests a progression where each level can only be achieved after the levels that come before are fulfilled. For example, the first level in Maslow's hierarchy is physiological needs. These are the bare necessities for a person's survival and include food, water, warmth, and shelter. It's reasonable to argue that if you're hungry and cold, it's going to be hard to think about anything else. You might have experienced this if you've attended a long, drawn-out meeting before lunch. It's hard to think about anything besides food. We all have a physiological need that we need to meet before we can focus on work. And if we don't have money, it's next to impossible to feel safe, which is something I experienced when I was young and can attest to.

According to Maslow, we must first satisfy the first four fundamental needs—physiological, safety, love and belonging, and esteem—before we can achieve a true sense of freedom in life and engage in self-actualization, which involves realizing our potential and contributing to others.

I realized that Maslow's first level—the physiological needs layer—also has many layers. To achieve physiological needs, we pretty much need another hierarchy altogether. To fulfill them, there is so much a person needs to know and do. We need to know what foods to eat, how to move and rest our body, and how to have healthy thoughts (because our brain is also part of our body).

There are five areas we know we need to focus on to stay healthy: nutrition, stress, fitness, sleep, and purpose. And managing these five is a job that's lifelong and requires daily focus. So, putting them into a model and breaking them down like Maslow did is one way to keep them in focus and ensure we are doing what we need to do to cover our health bases. Like Maslow's approach, there is a sequence to it, too, whereby we will struggle to achieve one area if another has not been met.

Borrowing cheekily from Maslow, I call it the Hierarchy of Longevity.

The Hierarchy of Longevity

The Hierarchy of Longevity (Figure 5.2) is a framework that makes knowing what to do to stay healthy simpler. It also defines the five health activities we all need to focus on and places them in a logical sequence.

Figure 5.2—The Hierarchy of Longevity

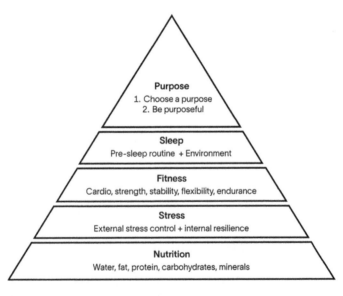

The Hierarchy of Longevity

Purpose
1. Choose a purpose
2. Be purposeful

Sleep
Pre-sleep routine + Environment

Fitness
Cardio, strength, stability, flexibility, endurance

Stress
External stress control + internal resilience

Nutrition
Water, fat, protein, carbohydrates, minerals

The Hierarchy of Longevity helps prioritize the actions we need to take in our life to optimize our health.

Let's look at each level and how they are interrelated, starting with nutrition.

1. Nutrition

The base of the Hierarchy of Longevity starts with nutrition. If you don't have the right fuel in your body, nothing matters. And that's why at Viome, we started there.

Imagine your body is a high-performance car; let's say a Ferrari. Now, think about the kind of fuel you're putting into this magnificent machine. If you fill it up with the wrong type of gas—like low-octane fuel when it needs a high-octane formulation—you'll have a sports car that may look slick but goes putt-putt, not vroom vroom. It would be a herky, jerky mess. So are you if you eat food low in essential nutrients and high in sugar, salt, and fat. Your system is going to knock and ping, and you'll never get very far in life.

Eating nutritious food is the foundation of health. It underpins all of the body's processes, and if there are insufficient nutrients available to your body, it can't function optimally. Without it, progressing up the hierarchy is challenging and potentially impossible. As you learned in the previous chapters, there is no such thing as universal healthy food or universal healthy supplements.

Your body and microbiome are unique to you. It changes when you change your diet and lifestyle. Stress also impacts your microbiome, and so does lack of sleep and exercise. And so, you have to constantly adapt your nutrition to your changing body. That's why we recommend that you test every six months to fine-tune your health for living healthier, longer.

> **My routine:**
> I personally follow the Viome food guidance and eliminate my "avoid" foods and eat my "enjoy" and "superfoods." More importantly, I take my supplements, gut biotics, and oral biotics religiously. I now have more energy than I did a decade ago, I have lost 20 lbs, and I have no brain fog and no memory issues at the age of 65. I love every minute of my life.

An undernourished body is less resilient to stress, so reaching level 2 of the hierarchy becomes more challenging if you have a nutritional deficiency.[120] You must also be strong and have optimal energy to train your body and keep it fit to reach level 3.[121] Sleep at level 4 becomes difficult too.[122] You might snooze too long because your body is malnourished. Certainly, if your brain and body lack nutrients, you won't be thinking about purpose (level 5). So, it is important to nourish the body to properly achieve the rest of the hierarchy for complete health.

2. Stress Management

The next level of the hierarchy is stress management. If your nutrition needs are not met, dealing with stress is going to be difficult. Without proper nutrition, the human body is less resilient to stress.

Our body's stress response saved us from predators in ancient times by initiating a fight or flight response when, say, a hungry predator showed up in our encampment. Upon detecting a threat, a part of the brain known as the hypothalamus activates an alert. This triggers a rush of hormones like adrenaline and cortisol into the bloodstream.[123]

Adrenaline accelerates your heart rate, elevates your blood pressure, and boosts your energy levels. Meanwhile, cortisol, a stress hormone, raises the levels of glucose (sugar) in your bloodstream, improves how your brain uses the glucose, and enhances the body's ability to repair tissues. Additionally, cortisol slows biological processes that are non-critical at the moment. It changes the immune system response and deprioritizes digestive, reproductive, and growth systems. This sophisticated emergency alert system also interacts with parts of the brain responsible for managing mood, motivation, and fear.[124]

Typically, the body's stress response is automatic. It deactivates once an immediate threat has subsided. Hormone levels normalize as adrenaline and cortisol diminish, restoring heart rate and blood pressure to their usual meter, and all bodily functions resume their normal state.[125]

If the body is under frequent or even constant stress and this automatic response fires frequently, its defensive processes never fully reset. That can cause health issues over the long term. Prolonged activation of the stress response system, coupled with excessive exposure to cortisol and other stress hormones, can disturb virtually every physiological process in the body. The by-product? Potentially, a multitude of health issues, from anxiety to depression to digestive disturbances and headaches to major issues like obesity, heart disease, and cancer.[126]

Today, there are no lurking tigers in the suburbs, but we live in a time when we are constantly under stress from other forces. The boss at work stresses us out. We go home, and our spouse spikes our cortisol with their spending on whatever caught their fancy at the mall. We navigate frustrating traffic jams and suffer yammering doomsayers on the news. And we self-diminish our-selves for being less than whatever we think we should be, comparing ourselves unrealistically to whatever we see in social feeds, the media, or across the fence. Our bodies are constantly in a fight-or-flight response. No wonder we can't digest our food. No wonder we get sick. Stress lowers immune system response.

Our best "treatments" for stress are many simple, time-honored rituals. With new technological tools, we have learned the science of why many traditional techniques work. For instance, in many religions, it is a tradition to pray before eating. Saying grace eases us out of stress and has us focus on the plate of food in front of us. In recent years, meditation has also become mainstream. Pausing helps switch the body from a sym-pathetic mode into a parasympathetic mode to regain optimal function.[127]

We're also seeing other age-old techniques, such as breathwork, sound baths, and forest bathing, becoming more commonplace. It's important to do more of the things you enjoy, like spending time with people you like, being with friends, doing things you love, reading books, or doing what brings joy into your life. And that reduces your stress, and that helps you live longer. So laugh as they say.

My routine:

I don't let anything or anyone stress me. I am the only one who causes stress to myself, and no one else has that power over me. Other people and stressful environments can be a trigger, but we are the ones that get ourselves stressed. I constantly remind myself that "it is what is" and "it will be what will be." There are

> only two types of situations in the world. One where it's out of my control, and that's when I simply take a deep breath and believe in the Universe, and I say to myself it will be what will be, and I no longer worry about it. The second is where it's in my control. In this situation, I do the best I possibly can, and then I trust the Universe, and I say to myself that I have done the best I can, and it will be what will be.

You also have to have faith in the Universe (or you may choose to call it God) that everything that's happening is for your good. As a matter of fact, I prefer to not categorize anything that's happening as good or bad. They just are. We all have experienced moments that seemed bad but turned out to be good in our own lives. A breakup that we thought was the worst thing that could have happened looks like a gift when you find someone you fall head over heels for.

Staying fit also helps with stress response, so movement is another activity we can all engage in more. It's also the third level of the Hierarchy of Longevity.

3. Movement

A critical piece of the health puzzle is movement. Why not call it exercise or fitness? I use the word "movement" because staying in motion and moving our bodies is extremely important for health, and it is inclusive and applicable for all ages.[128]

If you exercise, then certainly that is considered movement and fits into this. By all means, go to the gym, swim, bike, run, and play sports. But the point in calling it movement is that we all need to get in motion! Movement should be incorporated into your day whenever possible. Walk when you talk on the phone. Move yourself to the office coffee machine. Get off the couch or get away from your office chair and move your body as often as you can; you'll improve your health in the process.

We also know that strength training becomes extremely important as we age. Without it, the body loses muscle mass, connective tissue diminishes, and bone becomes less dense.[129] As we get older, we want to avoid losing muscle. Broken bones are one of the leading causes of early death. Many seniors have a higher risk of death up to ten years after an injury.[130] And many injuries lead to other adverse health events.

Exercises for strength don't need to be complicated. We can use body weight to build muscle very effectively. Exercises like squats, planks, and push-ups are activities we can all do that don't require equipment. There are basic exercises we can all do using our body as weight to build muscle. If we hike, we build those leg muscles. We can do yoga anywhere, anytime.

My routine:

You don't need to become a gym rat spending hours at the gym lifting weights. I walk fast, at least five miles a day (uphill most days), and I do strength training two to three times per week using body weight when I am traveling or using gym weights when I am at home.

Now, when you have engaged in enough movement, sleep quality is improved, and that is level four.

4. Sleep

When it comes to sleep, like most areas of life, quality matters more than quantity. People get too hung up on getting eight hours of shut-eye. Less is ok if you are getting enough time in each of the three sleep phases. Here is what we know from a scientific standpoint we should target:

- Deep sleep: One hour and fifteen minutes.
- Rapid Eye Movement (REM): An hour and a half of REM sleep.
- Light sleep: The rest of the night.

During deep sleep, the body repairs itself, strengthens the immune system, and improves bone structure and muscle. The phase that follows is known as Rapid Eye Movement (REM) and is characterized by rapid movement of the eyes, increased brain activity, paralysis of major muscles, and vivid dreaming.[131]

From an early age, my parents, who are followers of Jainism, taught me to avoid eating or drinking three to four hours before bedtime. Their religious practice prohibits eating after sunset. For a long time, I questioned the reason behind this. Eventually, I discovered there's a scientific basis for it: eating just before bed can significantly impair sleep quality.[132]

So, focus on getting at least 1.5-2 hours of REM sleep, 1.25-1.5 hours of deep sleep, and 2.5-3 hours of light sleep. Some people are able to get this in six hours, and that's amazing. Some need seven hours, and others need eight hours to get this quality of sleep. Again, it's the quality of sleep and not the quantity of sleep that matters. You also want the heart rate to be low when you are sleeping for great recovery the next day.

My routine:

I measure my sleep with a smart ring and mattress. Both of them track the various stages of sleep, my heart rate when I am sleeping, and my heart rate variability. I eat dinner early and I avoid eating anything else at least three hours before my bedtime, which is usually 9 pm. I generally don't drink any alcohol in the evening. As a matter of fact, I hardly drink alcohol at all because it disrupts my sleep. I also avoid caffeinated beverages after 3 pm. In the morning, I get up between 4–5 am, so I get an average of about seven or eight hours of sleep each night. As for sleep stages, I get 1.5 hours of REM sleep, 1.25 hours of deep sleep, and 3 hours of light sleep. There are nights I have to entertain and my sleep routine is disrupted, but I try to minimize those days.

Once you have developed healthy sleep habits, you'll find it easier to start your morning and maintain your energy throughout the day. A human who eats the right nutrients, has low stress, moves often, and sleeps well is well primed to engage in pursuits that make them happy and fulfilled. So, let's talk about purpose.

5. Purpose

If you wake up in the morning and don't jump out of bed excited and enthusiastic for the coming day, it's a sign you're not living purposefully.

Becoming well-rested primes you for a busy and fulfilling day and makes it physiologically easier to engage with life. When you have no purpose, it's a problem because living a purposeful life is key to optimal health and longevity. In fact, purpose is a catalyst for excellent health for five reasons:

1. Accomplishing ambitious goals requires energy and vitality, so we're naturally more inclined to make healthier choices.[133]
2. People with a sense of purpose tend to experience less stress, enjoy higher levels of fulfillment, and have more energy.[134]
3. Having a purpose equips us to handle stress more effectively. It encourages us to take more time to unwind, meditate, and enjoy quiet moments.[135]
4. Resistance to tasks lessens when our attention is centered on a significant goal. Challenges appear less intimidating, making every obstacle more manageable.[136]
5. Others with the same purpose are drawn to us, and we build stronger relationships. It's not possible to achieve any major purpose without a team of people around you.

Not surprisingly, many longevity studies have found a significant connection between having a purpose and physical health, including longer lifespans.[137] So, although purpose is the fifth and top layer on the Hierarchy of Longevity, it may arguably be the most critical aspect.

Live a life of purpose. Seek meaning in what you are doing. If you are a bus driver, relate to your job not as a driver of a large vehicle but as someone who enables thousands of people to get to work, to see their family, to go to their place of worship, and to live their lives. You make that possible. If you are a server at a restaurant, relate to your role as making it possible for people to eat delicious food that fuels their bodies and gives them a break from their kitchens. If you are a janitor, don't relate to yourself as just a cleaner but as someone who brings hygiene and health to the world. All these jobs are important and serve the public and the common good.

Ask yourself what you are willing to die for and live for it. What are you willing to dedicate your life to solving and then dedicate your life to doing it? Another way to look at this is to ask yourself what you would do if you had all the money you need and a great family. Now, do that, and you will get all the money you need, and you will build a great family because you have a purpose in life.

This is just a snapshot of how to approach purpose to help you start thinking about it in the context of the Hierarchy of Longevity. It is so important that I explore it at a deeper level in the next chapter.

My routine:

For me, I live a life of purpose. Each decade, I choose a new obsession to pursue. I find a big problem to tackle and spend every minute of my free time learning about it. Each month, I read three to four books and hundreds of research reports. My reading list is very broad and includes everything from inspirational biographies to learning about cancer to biocentrism. I read about quantum theory and wonder if we are living in a simulation. I read about why we age to how we age and wonder how we can increase the healthspan of humanity. Reading about a variety of diverse subjects allows you to look at the problem from various perspectives and potential solutions that may not be obvious to experts in the field.

The Hierarchy of Longevity is a worthwhile model for health, but it becomes far more useful when you know how to apply it to you. Where it starts to have utility is when you can take each area of the model and evaluate how its components apply to *your body*. To achieve this, we need to *measure* where we are within each layer of the hierarchy and then apply actions that improve the result. Let's look at that next.

Measure, Take Action, Repeat

Have you ever noticed how many experts make pronouncements on how their health solution is easy to follow and will help us stay thinner, younger, and more vibrant? Think about the avalanche of health messaging you see in the media or on the Internet. We are told to take an infrared sauna because it will make us younger. Or longevity drugs like Metformin or Rapamycin will help us live longer. We should also gorge on guacamole because, say the diet gurus, avocados are superfoods. And plant-based eating is better. No, wait, keto is best. And hold on, here comes the jackfruit diet, the coriander diet, or some other such nonsense.

And how about exercise? Some say it's more important than nutrition. Others say we don't need much if we're smart about it. Get 10,000 steps in per day, but be careful you don't overdo it and tear your meniscus. But definitely get your heart rate up, or you may as well stay on the couch. Sleep, but not too much. Stressed? Mediate! And so on.

Everyone has *the* solution, yet no one has a definitive answer to curing what ails us. Every time there is a new health fad, we all pay attention because our brains crave simple solutions. That's why people latch onto the latest quick fixes with the hope that they will be a cure-all and give us impeccable health and a long life.

So, what should we do? Who is right? There is no quick answer, no single magic pill or device. And certainly, there is no one single diet we should all eat for optimal health. That's because we are all unique. So, it is not possible to find one single magical quick fix that will solve the health puzzle for all of us in one go.

Yet, there is a way forward. What if I told you there is an extremely smart entity out there that knows exactly what you need to live a long and healthy life free of disease and dysfunction? It is a hyper-intelligent genius, and it knows everything that will ever be needed to keep you healthy, disease-free, and living for a very long time.

No, it's not AI. Or an app. Or your mother. That one thing is you—*You!* Or, more specifically, your body and the biological intelligence that runs within you and knows you best. It is your first line of defense against tiny invaders that want to break into your system and wreak havoc. It knows what foods make you feel great, and it also knows which ones are not ideal.

When you experience hunger, thirst, sleepiness, or feel aroused, that is a message from your body to your brain (or rather the "conscious" you) to eat, drink, sleep, or cuddle up to a mate. And when those needs become urgent, your body dials up the signals making them louder and more uncomfortable so that you can't ignore them.

Equally efficient is the pain mechanism. Your body reports crises that need immediate attention with aches, soreness, and increasingly acute pain to indicate an injury or damage that needs to be remedied. Pain is a signal to stop and assess and, if needed, seek help. Our bodies are resilient. If there are small deficiencies within its systems, it copes by itself. Its self-management capabilities are automatic, so at the biological level, it will use whatever resources are available to compensate for any shortcomings. It's clever that way.

Your body constantly communicates in a language we don't fully understand, sending non-urgent messages that could help you prevent disease and extend your life. That's why we created Viome: to help you decode these messages transmitted through RNA so we can address underlying issues before they escalate into symptoms or diseases. Our bodies are designed to maintain homeostasis or balance. When they break down due to poor maintenance, they enter a state of "dis-ease," which we call disease.

For some people, that might mean that they may look and even feel mostly healthy for decades, and then one day–BOOM!–they suffer a massive coronary and drop dead where they stand. Perhaps you might have trouble walking up the stairs sometimes or get mentally or physically fatigued on a particularly intense day. Poor nutrition will also lead to low energy and, eventually, a low mood. Your body might issue clues along the way, but in some regards, it has no early warning messaging system, at least none that makes us aware, for example, that your cholesterol is high thanks to your donut-rich diet. For the first thousand (or so) donuts you eat in your life, it will largely remain silent and tolerant of the onslaught of all that fried, sugary dough that you are freight training into your gut.

All is not lost, however. We now have the technology to collect personalized data so we can understand what's happening inside each of us with higher fidelity than ever before. The data we can collect has become so advanced that, when interpreted, it can expose a problem long before the body communicates a developing disease state.

The bottom line is: You have been the missing part in your health equation. Once you know what you—your body—needs and the strategies that work, figuring out what to do to counteract unwanted states and stay healthy becomes easy.

You have been the missing part in your health equation.

So, how do you put that into practice? You go back to the Hierarchy of Longevity, but instead of evaluating each level subjectively, as in, "I think I eat nutritiously because I feel pretty good," you use empirical knowledge, as in: "I know I eat well because I have collected data from my body that proves it."

The Youth Formula

So, where's the formula we promised in this book? How do you stay biologically young and healthy and extend your life for as long as possible?

You use the Youth Formula, which is as follows:

$$f(\text{Knowledge} + \text{You}^{\text{Technology}}) = \text{Optimized Health Behaviors} \rightarrow \text{Health and Longevity}$$

Let's simplify the equation.

Knowledge: This is all the accumulated human health knowledge that scientists have learned over time. It represents our current scientific understanding and information about health, nutrition, genetics, and aging. The Hierarchy of Longevity is a handy distillation of that knowledge in a simplified framework that makes it easier to digest and less daunting to use.

You^{Technology}: You to the power of technology means measuring your body using technology tools to gain data points you can monitor. It is using tools like Viome's Full Body Intelligence Test and other AI-driven health technologies that tailor recommendations and interventions based on individual data.

The f is short for "function". In a formula, it is like a tool: it takes an input, follows a rule to process it, and provides an answer.

Using plain English and making it simple, here's what it all means: When you take what we know about human health and combine it with high-resolution data from your body using measurement technology, you can more accurately calculate the actions you need to take to live a long, healthy, life.

Let's put this formula into action so you can see it applied.

Your Roadmap for Longevity

Applying the Youth Formula, we need to measure our bodies as it applies to each element of the Hierarchy of Longevity so that we can design new actions to improve our results for each area.

Here is how this looks, starting with nutrition. You'll see that if you use the formula and apply it to what you eat, you can nourish your body more effectively.

Nutrition 2.0

With nutrition, we have known for centuries that we need the following six nutritional components to function:[138]

1. Water
2. Protein
3. Fat
4. Carbohydrates
5. Vitamins
6. Minerals

Of course, how much of each of these elements we need varies by person. The percentage of each component is determined by height, weight, age, sex, and health goals.

However, more recently, we have learned that biochemical individuality, which is what each person's body needs at a molecular level to thrive, matters too. This is where knowing what to eat has become more accurate and where Viome, as you know, has innovated. By using AI on data collected from test kit samples, we can process massive datasets to determine whether what a person eats is optimally nutritious for ideal health.

AI learns as it processes more data, so with every sample processed, we reduce errors, incorrect information, bias, and subjectivity. Our success continues to get us closer to preventing chronic diseases and can help slow down aging by using the measurements we make to adjust what we eat. In this process, we are continuously learning and improving, and accuracy gets better every day with each sample we process.

In doing so, we take the information from your data and assess it across hundreds of foods to target the best food choices for you. Viome tests allow us to provide personalized food lists with precise information about each food and why your body needs it based on data. What we've been able to do is this:

Figure 5.3—How Viome science leads to food recommendations

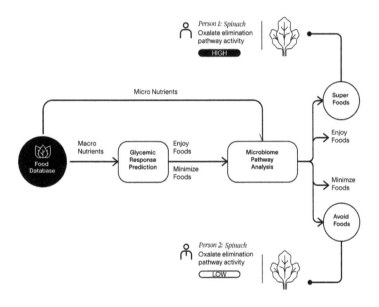

Viome's food database contains 300 foods that are sorted by analyzing stool, saliva, and blood samples based on criteria of glycemic response and microbiome pathway analysis to create personalized food recommendations.

Macronutrients from each food are used to precisely determine the glycemic response of the food within each individual. Micronutrients are evaluated in the context of a collection of pathway activities, such as butyrate production, oxalate elimination, and sulfide production.

All this information is used to determine whether each food is a superfood, a food to enjoy, minimize, or avoid for a specific individual whose data we analyze. We use a similar method for determining supplement ingredient recommendations.

Nutrition science has undergone a paradigm shift where the key to eating for health is to consume exactly what each body needs, ensuring we get the molecular components for optimum health. As an approach, think about Nutrition 2.0, as depicted in Figure 5.4.

Figure 5.4—The Nutrition 2.0 Approach

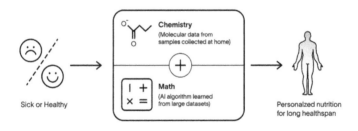

Nutrition 2.0 is the process of calculating which foods are necessary for each person to ensure optimum health and longevity.

What we've learned is that there is no one-size-fits-all solution. Certain foods are not good for some people. *Biochemical individuality* is key. This is why no one diet is universally ideal for everyone.

Historically, eating for biochemical individuality hasn't been easy because we haven't had the tools available to make this process simple and affordable. For those of you who went to primary school several decades ago, you might have wondered why the food pyramid (or "MyPlate" as it is called in the U.S. today) has changed over the years. Food science continues to evolve, necessitating new guidelines. We were once advised that carbohydrates were the most important food to eat! Nowadays, the guideline recommends a balanced approach between fruit, vegetables, grains, protein, and dairy (and plant-based alternatives). Interestingly, consuming high carbs made sense during World War II when soldiers were too thin and needed fattening up.[139]

To make health simpler, governments establish guidelines like the food pyramid to guide the populace toward a healthier life. The U.S. food pyramid is no longer a pyramid. It's now a plate. Canada also has a food guide. Australia has a food pyramid, and China, interestingly enough, has a food guide pagoda.[140]

But we've debunked this idea that there are universal health foods for all. When it comes to everything we eat, from foods and beverages to supplements, eating right means eating for what your body needs. Without the right fuel in the body, nothing matters.

Recommended measurement action:

Measure your body's response to the food you eat using tools like the ones Viome has developed. Adapt your eating habits for optimal health. Supplement where needed. Retest as you go.

You can also compare your response to certain foods to a friend or partner's response. Notice differences in foods that make you feel energized, alert, bloated, or fatigued. This highlights individual variability. You will find that foods affect you differently.

Next, let's look at how this applies to how we manage stress.

Be Resilient

Stress isn't bad and avoiding stress altogether is not possible. Still, for optimal health, we need to find ways to deal with stress in proactive, positive ways.

Stress management is a balancing act. If you want to manage stress effectively, there are two areas that require constant attention and practice.[141]

1. External stimulus control
2. Internal resilience training

External stimulus control is about controlling our environments so we don't put ourselves into situations where we are exposed to excessive stress. For example, let's say that a person is in a bad relationship or marriage that causes constant levels of stress because of conflict, disharmony, or general unhappiness. In this case, there are new actions that can be taken to minimize stress levels. They could get rid of the root cause of the stress by leaving the relationship, or they could work to improve the relationship by attending counseling sessions in an effort to resolve conflict and improve communication.[142] Regardless of the remedy chosen, the person is actively minimizing their stress by taking control of their external environment.

Internal resilience training is about how well we control stress when it occurs. Since we can't eliminate all stress in our lives, learning coping mechanisms is important. This can be complicated because there is both a physiological and a mindset component to stress. One tried and true technique when stress occurs is to pause any activity, where possible, and quiet the mind or engage in an activity that brings us joy. A caveat here, though: don't do this on the highway at 60 mph unless you can find a way to do it safely.[143]

Sometimes, you can reduce stress by being with people you like to spend time with or finding pleasure in simple things that you love to do. Perhaps you like reading. If so, read more books (perhaps ones by an entrepreneur named Naveen). Other common stress-reduction activities range from mindfulness practices to therapeutic techniques to mental resilience training regimes.

Also, keep in mind that there are nutrients and foods that can support your health (again, why nutrition comes first on the hierarchy). For example, nutrients like magnesium and vitamin B6 become depleted in times of stress.[144] Foods containing caffeine or alcohol can exacerbate stress.[145] Foods high in DHA/EPA, probiotic-rich foods, and fiber-rich foods are all great for supporting stress.[146]

While there are mindset tools and techniques we know work for everyone, it's a matter of testing and learning what works for you. Here is what we know works for most people, and it is backed with scientific data to show these are effective stress reduction approaches.

External stimulus control:

- Avoid toxic environments
- Don't engage in high-risk situations where the reward is low
- Manage finances

Internal resilience training:

- Eat a precision diet
- Test for toxins—another type of anti-nutrient we may not realize is impacting our body

- Optimize your movement and sleep
- Engage in recovery/resilience practices for the body: sauna, bath or hot tub, massage, cold plunges, deprivation tanks
- Enjoy meditation and mindfulness practices
- Engage in hobbies
- Spend time in nature. Forest bathing, or Shinrin-yoku, is a research-backed tool for stress management
- Learn metacognitive practices—these are practices that allow us to think about our thinking and shift perspective. They range from traditional cognitive behavior (CBT) and dialectic therapies (DBT) to neuro-linguistic programming (NLP) to less traditional mindset frameworks
- Spend time with people who make you feel good

A body that is not under major stress has more attention and energy to put into exercise because it is not using massive amounts of energy to pump out cortisol.[147] So, now you can move and train your body and experience superior benefits.

Recommended measurement action:

Measure your stress levels with a smartwatch. A measurement called Heart Rate Variability (HRV) can show imbalances in your autonomic nervous system, which can indicate your stress levels. Your heart rate variability is determined by the balance between the responses in your sympathetic and parasympathetic nervous systems. There are a variety of apps that can measure HRV and fire alerts where stress levels appear to be spiking. Search for HRV measuring tools on your mobile device's app store.[148]

Keep Moving

When it comes to movement, we know that the human body benefits from the following five forms of movement[149]:

1. **Cardiovascular:** Activities that raise and maintain an elevated heart rate over the duration of the exercise. Vigorous walking, jogging, or running are good examples, but you could ride a bike, go for a long swim, or engage in any exercises that raise your heart rate for 30 to 60 minutes at a time.

2. **Strength training:** Lift weights to build muscle mass. You don't need to go to the gym and pump iron. Pushups, squats, and other exercises that lift your own body weight are good choices. So is yoga, gardening, or any other activity that requires you to lift objects repeatedly.

3. **Endurance:** When moving, work on your ability to extend how you can maintain the effort. Some people walk or run every day and, on the weekend, choose a longer walk or run to help develop their endurance.

4. **Flexibility:** Stretch your muscles so they are loose and limber. Simple stretching exercises are easy to find on the Internet. Yoga and Pilates are also good for enhancing flexibility.

5. **Stability:** Engage the muscles that stabilize your body and help you balance. Planks, balancing, and squats are all good stability exercises.

Which area to focus on should be determined by *what your body needs*. For this you need to know your baseline physical state of health. It will help you determine what exercises to do and for what duration.

So, how often should you exercise? You do not need to become a gym rat and spend hours pumping iron. It is a lifestyle! It is simply about making sure that you move every day for 30 to 45 minutes in a way that gets your heart rate up. Move every hour if you can. I like to walk four or five miles each day. If I have a meeting with a colleague, I like to walk and talk. If I need a break, I walk down the street near my office and get tea. If you build habits like that into your day, you will be in a good place. Once you've built that habit, you'll feel better. You'll manage stress better, and you will certainly start to sleep better, too.

Recommended measurement action:

Wearable fitness technologies like smartwatches or fitness trackers can monitor your daily steps and set thresholds you'd like to meet. They can also calculate calorie burn and heart rate levels during movement and provide daily reports on your efforts. That said, you don't need a smart gadget to measure your effort; you can certainly do it manually with a notebook and pencil, but the tech tools available are increasingly affordable and can be had for under $100 and some even lower than $50. Some mobile phones will even track your steps by measuring motion. Open the health app that comes with your phone and explore it. You'll be surprised at what it already tracks, including, in most cases, your sleep patterns.

Sleep Success

According to sleep science, how much shut-eye we need varies by human, but it is safe to say we all need 1 to 2 hours of deep sleep. Most people go through two types of sleep in each cycle:

- o One stage of rapid eye movement (REM) and
- o Three stages of non-rapid eye movement (NREM)
  - Light (N1)
  - Deep (N2)
  - Deeper sleep (N3)

A person cycles through these stages 4–5 times every night. According to experts, the stages cycle in this order: N1, N2, N3, N2, REM. Each cycle lasts around 90 to 110 minutes. The first REM stage is short, but as sleep progresses, it gets longer compared with NREM.[150]

There are simple measures we can all take to get our best night's sleep, but again, personalization is key. Do what works for you, although these six techniques work for most.[151]

1. Sleep in a dark room
2. Avoid alcohol and large meals before sleep
3. Have a safe, comfortable place to sleep
4. Avoid exposure to bright light before sleep
5. Ensure we have a quiet sleep environment
6. Sleep in a room with a temperature of between 60 and 67°F (15.6 and 19.4°C)

Obviously, a sleep environment is a personal choice, but if you're struggling to achieve restful sleep, you can make adjustments based on these techniques.

Recommended measurement:

Basic sleep-tracking technology is built into most mobile phone health apps. A smartwatch or fitness tracker can track sleep cycles based on movement, heart rate, and other indicators. There are also smart beds and sleep sensors that slip under your mattress and report your night's sleep to a mobile device or computer.

And, of course, sleeping is always better if you have a purpose to wake up to!

Intentional Living

Finding (and keeping) a purpose in life differs between each person, of course, but there are two practices that work for everyone. They are:

1. Pursuing a moonshot
2. Being purposeful

We will spend some time in the final chapter on these two approaches because it requires a more in-depth discussion. However, the key to finding a purpose is to devise a goal you want to pursue. You can also bring purpose to any given moment by seeing it from a new perspective. The simplest way to do that is to consider what you want in life and set goals and parameters so the intangibility of life can be measured. It's the only way to know where you are going and if you are moving forward or stagnating.

Purpose has a fascinating reverberating effect on the other areas. If a person loses their purpose in life, health can start to wane. I noticed that with my dad. Once he retired, he lost his purpose, and I believe that contributed to the decline in his health.

So, I am happy to see a slightly different trajectory for my mom. Despite the death of my dad, her husband, she has refocused her life by staying busy with volunteer work in her community. Helping her enjoy life and staying healthy is also meaningful for me, and it fits nicely into my purpose.

Recommended measurement action:

Measuring your purpose in life is a little more difficult than it is with the other layers of the hierarchy because it is more subjective. That said, you can measure it by asking yourself questions and tracking your responses. Here are some of my favorites:

- What are you willing to die for so you can live for it?
- What matters to you in your life?
- When you wake up in the morning, do you jump out of bed? If you don't jump out of bed, then what could you do that will make you want to?

You can also visit TheYouthFormula.com for more tools to help you with your purpose. Whatever you do, track your answers, make changes, and ask the questions again. It will help you measure your purpose, and with a well-defined purpose, you will be healthier for it. It's a critical aspect of health, and it is so important that we will come back to this topic in the final chapter.

What about Your Mom, Naveen?

Before we leave this chapter, I thought I would leave you with a little inspiration from my mother, who is doing rather well in the five areas of health.

Every six months, my mom tests her microbiome to ensure that she is eating the nutrients her body needs to stay balanced and avoid any pre-disease states that may be lurking in her system. Her precise eating habits have improved her health, and she also takes the recommended custom supplements Viome makes for her.

She also continues to master all the other areas of the Hierarchy of Longevity. When it comes to managing stress, she really doesn't have much. When I ask her about it, she says, "What is there for me to worry about? My children are doing fine. I am fine. I don't have anything to stress about."

Sleep has never been an issue; she's always been a good sleeper. Following the Jainism tradition, she never eats after sundown. She always sleeps well and wakes to greet the sunrise.

When it comes to exercise, she doesn't go to the gym, but she does move every day. She is in constant motion and busies herself with the matters of the day. And she certainly needs to because she's focused on a purpose; she does a lot of spiritual work, including meditation and praying. Her context for life is that nothing is scarce. And although she is retired, she has a greater purpose. She is building a charitable foundation that will fund a new temple for her spiritual community.

I have watched her get better and better in each of the five areas. She is an inspiration, and if she keeps going, I believe she will make it to 106 like my great-grandmother or beyond. So, let's all take some inspiration from her. If we all follow similar habits, like the superagers who have come before us, we can remain in peak shape as we age.

The Mindset Shift

If you take one insight from this chapter, let it be this...

Your body signals what it needs to avoid aging and decline.

By using tools to collect data about your body, you will know what it needs and what you need to do to stay healthy.

Health is personal. Each body needs different things at different times to stay healthy.

Key Insights

- Lifestyle matters more than genetics in the pursuit of health and longevity.
- There are five key areas that require constant attention and they are: 1) nutrition, 2) stress management, 3) movement, 4) sleep, and 5) purpose.
- The Hierarchy of Longevity is a model that demonstrates there is a sequence to the five areas, where it gets harder to achieve each level if the one before needs attention.
- The only way to know if you are succeeding in any aspect of health is to measure it.

- Once upon a time, we didn't have tools that would allow us to gain sophisticated insights about our bodies. Today, we do, and they will get more sophisticated over time.
- We can use the Hierarchy of Longevity like a menu by adding universal scientific perimeters to each layer, track what we need, and factor our body's data against health fundamentals.
- f (Knowledge + You^{Technology}) = Optimized Health Behaviors → Health and Longevity is a formula we can all use to stay healthy
- Nutrition 2.0 is how we should eat to stay healthy. It's about considering the molecular components of food and what our body needs on a molecular level, then eating in accordance. This is where Viome has innovated.
- Success with managing stress is about: 1) External stimulus control and 2) internal resilience training.
- Movement should be a constant focus. Staying fit is less about being a gym rat and more about frequent, intentional movement. Strength training becomes more important as we age.
- When it comes to sleep, think quality over quantity. We need about 1 to 2 hours of deep sleep every night.
- Purpose matters and helps us stay healthy. When we have a purpose, we want to continue living and thriving.
- What we need to do for our health and what works for each one of us is personal and changes over the course of our lives.

CHAPTER 6
WHAT'S YOUR CHOICE?

Only those who risk going too far can possibly find
out how far one can go.

—*T. S. Eliot*

Almost a decade ago, when I started Viome, my health was very different than it is today. My first biological age test showed my body was two years older than my chronological age. I was 57, with the body of a 59-year-old. I did not have a chronic disease or a major health issue, but I was beginning to feel the signs of age. I had an extra few inches around my belly, and I was experiencing digestive issues like acid reflux. I also had low energy, which was frustrating. Today, it is a very different story.

As I write this, I am 65, with a biological age of 52. The process to get here has been fairly simple. I have made numerous and persistent tweaks to my lifestyle. They took little effort, yet I now have excellent health. Every year, I get biologically younger, which my wife certainly has no problem with. I often say to her: *Anu, you cougar, you!* And then we laugh. She is getting younger, too.

I went from eating common "universally healthy foods" like spinach, avocado, and strawberries to eating my recommended superfoods and adjusting my diet according to my microbiome. I have also incorporated more activities into my day. My colleagues and I are committed to a walking meeting culture at Viome. We don't always meet across a boardroom table; we walk and talk when we can.

I have also become much more focused on downtime. I am an extremely busy CEO who loves what he does, but I wouldn't be able to do what I do if I wasn't fastidious about periods of rest. One of my favorite pastimes is hiking with family and friends. I enjoy being

If you have been conditioned to believe you must "grind it" to succeed, heed some advice from this wise old/young man: take downtime.

in nature on these walks and pausing to make a big deal about the critters we see in our path. Just last week, I was hiking with a group of friends near my home in the British Virgin Islands, and we saw a hermit crab that had scuttled about and hid in its shell when we got too close.

I am telling you this—especially for those who are also busy executives—because pausing and enjoying life not only fuels your soul but it benefits your business, too. If you have been conditioned to believe you must "grind it" to succeed, heed some advice from this wise old/young man: take downtime. I couldn't have built twelve successful businesses without it. Downtime allows for reflection, recalibration, and regeneration. It is the antidote to persistent and unyielding stress.

I have always prioritized sleep and purpose, but I have added more rigor to these areas of my life, too. As I've previously mentioned, I track my sleep using a sensor ring on my finger, an app on my phone, and a smart mattress pad. As my parents taught me, I never eat or drink two hours before my head hits the pillow each night. This really helps with my quality of sleep.

My journey has also reinforced the idea that living with purpose is crucial for fulfillment and empowerment in all aspects of my life, including my health. My work with Viome has further strengthened my commitment to mentor as many people as possible, helping them find their purpose and embark on missions that enhance lives. This is important to me. It is one of the many things that give me a reason to get up in the morning, and I find great satisfaction in it when I close my eyes at night.

Since 2017, I have reshaped my body. I've lost twenty-five pounds. I've shed fat, and I have maintained and grown my muscle mass by adding simple strength training exercises here and there. I now have almost zero visceral fat on my body. And I have much more energy than I ever had, which is wonderful! At 65, I'm just getting started. It is remarkable to live in a more vital body, yet become wiser as I chronologically age. I feel like a force to be reckoned with in this world. And I want this for everyone.

Developing a healthier body has also strengthened my conviction to help others understand the value of health and see that it is possible for themselves. This book is, of course, part of the mission, and I hope you will join me.

Forming a team at Viome has also proven to me, once again, that if you work with people who want to make a difference in the world, then anything is possible—even a mission as complex as aging and health. I do not doubt that one day, aging and the chronic diseases that come with it will no longer be a problem. As we each commit to a healthy body and life, we make it possible for not just ourselves but our children and grandchildren, too.

Taking the actions necessary to prioritize health and seeing the results for myself, my mother, and my colleagues has only cemented my resolve that it is possible for everyone.

The thing is, though, we need to *choose* it. And that might be the toughest step of all.

Believe It, Choose It

So, how do you choose to live a healthy life? It might sound simple, and perhaps it is, at its core. You make a choice, like: "I am going to be healthier, and that will result in me living longer and disease-free." And then… and then what?

No one can make the choice for you, although you might have been prodded—by your doctor, your spouse, your children, your extended family, or your friends— that you probably should do something to improve your health. They might have urged you to lose weight, to start exercising, or to eat better. Your bed partner might have mentioned that you snore. (*"Maybe it's sleep apnea! Isn't that dangerous?"*) And so on, ad nauseam. None of them can force you to choose better health. That's up to you.

So, choose! And if you choose not to do anything, so be it. Put this book back on the shelf, or better, give it to someone else.

If you make a choice to improve your health, well, good. Now we have more to talk about. Choosing health and a longer life puts you on a new path. It means you'll need to take on some new actions starting today. Here's the first action that will really help you.

Start by visualizing that your body is fit and vital. See yourself living the life you want with the body that helps, not hinders you. Do this often.

In the last chapter, we gave you two tools, a one-line formula, a simplification of *The Youth Formula*, which is as follows:

$$f(Knowledge + You^{Technology}) = Optimized\ Health\ Behaviors \rightarrow Health\ and\ Longevity$$

We also gave you the Hierarchy of Longevity, a framework that outlines the areas of your health to evaluate, measure, improve, and then re-measure. All this so you can track your progress.

It all sounds relatively simple so far, right? On Day 1, review each area of the hierarchy and determine where you are. Document some **You have to choose health every day.** initial measurements so you have a starting point for each area of the hierarchy. It is worth keeping track of each area in a notebook or on your computer in a spreadsheet or whatever works best for you.

On the second day, you'll need to choose your health again. Yes, again. Choosing is not a one-time thing. You have to choose health every day. Each day, you have multiple opportunities to act in new and healthful ways.

Here's an example. You are hungry or have that vague gnawing feeling that you want a nibble of something, maybe something sweet. There's a tub of ice cream in the freezer. It is your favorite. There is a fruit bowl nearby, too. And there are some nice sweet oranges in it. It's time to choose (again). Think about your commitment. Visualize your healthy body. Then it's easy to choose the orange.

Or here's another scenario: This time, you are at work. You have to discuss an issue with a colleague. You could go to a vacant room, sit and meet, or you can choose your health and suggest that the two of you walk and talk, perhaps toward the local coffee shop. If you walk at a leisurely but intentional pace, where you are not out of breath, but you are breathing harder, that's movement. Do that for around nine or ten minutes, and you'll log about half a mile, then walk back. That's a total of a mile. See how easy it is to walk a mile, even if you don't have time to "exercise."

One more example: For better sleep, put your phone away (or put it on "Do Not Disturb" or "Airplane Mode") before getting into bed and save that one last email you need to send for the morning. Go to bed. Put your head on the pillow. Close your eyes. It's a simple choice.

These are all small and almost insignificant actions. Yet, they will have a massive impact when you cluster them all together each and every day over a period of time. The choices are simple; the impact is massive.

Each time you make a choice to take an action that is positive for health and you get a payoff, your brain and body will want more. Often, it gets easier because, over time, you build habit loops and pathways in the body.

Also, surrounding yourself with supportive people is key. If those around you don't support you, it can be hard to stick to habits. For me, this has been easier with my Viome community, where we connect and motivate each other.

Expect Resistance from People and Institutions

There will be some friction in this endeavor. People are generally well-meaning, but sometimes they may try to sway you to their way of approaching health. Perhaps your colleague doesn't want to walk and talk. Perhaps your spouse wants to share a bowl of ice cream with you. It is all innocent, but your new habits might be confronting for people around you.

Your doctor or primary healthcare provider might not entirely agree with your new actions or your approach. Not perhaps about walking meetings or eating oranges instead of ice cream, but they may be dubious about new health technologies you want to use. Perhaps they want to refer you to a dietician in their office instead of using a personalized home kit to work on your nutrition. They mean well, but it may be counter to your new approach to using The Youth Formula. You to the power of old technology = yesterday's behaviors.

You to the power of old technology = yesterday's behaviors.

Remember, today's healthcare institutions have not caught up to the times. New innovations can take institutions years to adopt. Our healthcare systems and the cultures within them are not designed to help us defeat aging and avoid disease. When you are sick, insurance firms, pharmaceutical companies, and hospitals make money. No one makes money when you are well. This doesn't mean they are full of bad people who want you to be sick and live a shortened life. But their very existence relies on the fact that they treat symptoms of illness and alleviate the discomfort of decline. They are not motivated to prevent you from aging or getting sick. (And, I will pause here to say this is not true of all professional healthcare workers or all sectors of the healthcare system. There are exceptions.) But remember that the system was designed at an earlier time, so it can't possibly provide you with the newest thinking and strategies around improving your healthspan and reversing aging long before you get sick and decrepit.

To become really good at overriding the resistance, there are two things to consider. First, know this resistance is normal, and how you handle it is going to be critical to your success. Second, expect more of it because technology is on an exponential path, and it is going to arrive extremely quickly and with many new options in the coming years. Institutional healthcare will struggle to keep up. There will be intense and uncomfortable disruption. Meanwhile, outliers that adapt to it quickly, like you and me, will have to be ready for this because there are massive opportunities available within the disruption for people focused on their healthspan.

The other piece of wisdom that I want you to embrace is my guidance on how to find a strong purpose for yourself. It's the only way you will choose great health at times when it seems that the world is against you.

The rest of this chapter will train you how to do both of these things. Let's start with a deeper understanding of where the world is heading. There's a phenomenon you need to understand and take advantage of if you want great health. I call it the Opportunity Gap.

The Opportunity Gap

We live in a remarkable era, a period of rapid evolution driven by AI. It is a precursor to a mind-bending period of innovation where human capabilities are supercharged even further by accelerating technology. It may feel like we are characters in a science fiction novel, yet it will be science fact. I am talking about brain and biochips, AI-driven home diagnostic technologies, bio-printed organs and body parts, real-time health analytic sensors (think "smart toilets"), accelerated healing therapies, and medical robots.

This will all lead to a phenomenon some experts have described as "the gap," which I call the Opportunity Gap.[152]

> Technology is moving much faster than governments, the economy, and the establishment.

The Opportunity Gap is a metaphor that explains this moment in our history as humans when technology is moving much faster than governments, the economy, and the establishment, as well as societal institutions like education, religion, and the general status quo.

Figure 6.1—The rate of science and technology growth versus institutions

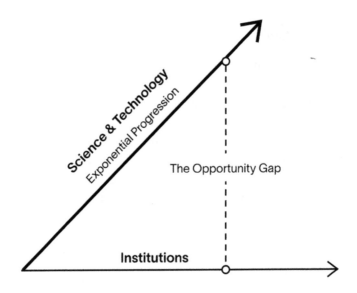

The Opportunity Gap exposes how technology outpaces societal institutions, such as government, education, healthcare, and religion.

Technology is growing at an exponential rate, which means that the rate of change is speeding up. The increasingly sophisticated tools included in that exponential improvement are driving access to better and more detailed personal health data.

Remember the part of The Youth Formula that is expressed as this:

$$You\ ^{Technology}$$

The "technology" variable in that part of the formula amplifies what we know about you. As it improves, the data about you gets better.

Let's use an example. If that technology is a microscope, it can reveal small structures in your body, and so your doctor might have once peered into it to discover a cell that is cancerous. Now fast forward and that technology is now an MRI scanner. The data about you and the cancer is amplified. An MRI can "see" cancer progression, tumor type, blood flow to a tumor, and so much more. That improved data informs new actions to take that can be lifesaving.

What happens when that technology gets even better than that? Like what we've done at Viome. We've combined genetic technology—metatranscriptomics—with AI to create a new tool, our AI engine that we call Vie. Vie has processed over a million data sets, and that has allowed us to make new connections and understand human health processes deeper than ever before. We can see pre-disease states that you can easily and affordably remedy (by eating differently) long before cancer can form.

Where is the medical system today in all this? It can use blood tests to detect some cancers. A doctor can also send you for an MRI, a technology invented in the 1970s (50 years ago!) that has evolved and become better over the decades. The latest generation of MRI is high-field MRI and functional MRI (fMRI) introduced in the last 20 to 30 years, which expanded the applications of MRI beyond anatomy into areas such as brain functionality and metabolic changes.[153]

But healthcare institutions—and perhaps your family doctor—have yet to adopt tools, for example, that we have developed at Viome. And, besides our technology, imagine all the other amazing cutting-edge technologies being developed today by entrepreneurs in the health sector that could help your doctor and hospitals serve you better. That can't happen with any velocity because institutions struggle to adapt and move quickly. Adoption of new tools, even if they are very useful and more effective than what is currently being used, takes time. Groups of people are not good at adapting and shifting behaviors quickly, especially if they've become used to a certain way of doing things. And the larger the group, the longer it can take for them to adopt and embrace anything new.

Think of it this way. On an individual level, if you need a new computer, you choose it and buy it. In a few days, it is on your desk. Not so for a hospital worker. They have to get it approved by their boss. Then, the IT department scopes approved technologies that will work with existing networks and ensure compatibility with specialty hospital software. It could take weeks, even months, before that new computer arrives on the worker's desk. Now, change the words "new computer" to "new MRI." The time between a decision to deployment becomes magnified.

Breakthroughs arrive faster than the time it takes for large groups to learn about, choose, and adopt them. This has always been the case. However, the difference today is that innovations are arriving so quickly that institutions can't keep up. And so the gap grows. While this might seem depressing and frustrating, there is also an intriguing upside. And this is why I don't just call it "the Gap." There is a massive opportunity in it, for anyone that is paying attention. That now includes you. This is why I call it the Opportunity Gap.

We have entered an era of unlimited opportunities where every person has more control over their lives. The power has shifted to the people—to *us*. We are experiencing what economist Thomas Friedman once predicted—the era of Globalization 3.0. He said that one day, individuals would have more power and control than governments and countries to enact major change.[154] That time is here today. This can have a massive impact on your ability to manage and optimize your health—to avoid disease and reverse aging.

Simply put, we cannot wait for institutions—be it the healthcare system, the government, or other social or cultural structures—to catch up. If we do, we will literally die waiting.

How to Use the Opportunity Gap

Let's get practical. Using the Opportunity Gap for improved health is simple. It simply requires that we stay aware of what is newly available or coming soon. Subscribe to health newsletters. Read science, technology, or health magazines. Use Google News to find keywords that you are interested in. Also, keep an eye on the business, health, and technology sections of your local online newspaper or news site. For example, a quick look at the *New York Times* Health section (on a weekday in April 2024, as this is written) reveals three headlines of note: *A.I. Could Spot Breast Cancer Earlier. Should You Pay for It? Should Alcoholic Beverages Have Cancer Warning Labels?* As well as, *How Does Alcohol Affect the Gut Microbiome?* All three are relevant to extending our healthspan.

So, what's coming? Keywords to keep an eye on include microbiome, longevity, robots, nanobots, bioengineering, and health home tests. I could go on, but you get the idea. Make your own list and take an interest in what pops up when you do web searches.

There are some very intriguing innovations coming soon, and they are worth tracking. Surgeons can already replace our knees, hips, and heart valves, among other body part replacements. The bioengineering work to create full replacements for heart, lungs, and other vital organs is underway. You may have heard that lab-grown steaks are in development. A steak is just cow muscle from various parts of the animal's body.

Similar technology will soon enable us to grow any organ from our cells and replace failing ones as they wear out. We may one day have nanorobots in our bodies that monitor and repair deficiencies, restoring healthy tissue. Then, what if we can download our memories and experiences and transfer them to a new biological body or non-biological body? Would that still be us? We will likely overcome the idea of death one day. It is a topic I am fascinated by.

Tools will become more personalized and affordable and accessible because of consumer demand, too. Eventually, there will be more integration of technology with our biology, redefining human capability. We will use innovations to enhance our physical and cognitive capacities. Today, we look at our smartphones to find the nearest plant-based restaurant or one with organic menu items. One day, it would be reasonable to imagine that we'll have chips in the brain to connect to the Internet. If the information we need is not top of mind, we will be able to summon it from the cloud. It will be one thought away.

Technological growth will lead to advances in every facet of well-being, offering new ways to treat diseases, streamline operations, and improve patient care. We are already seeing this in health where the era of precision health is here and growing. New tech and convergence are helping us create tools to learn more and stay healthier.

Our scientific understanding of the world around us is also ballooning in remarkable ways. Many experts use the word "disruption" because old ways of doing things are more rapidly being replaced by new and better methods. Adapting to these changes can seem difficult at times, and "disruption" may seem like a scary word. While it may be unnerving, disruption is also good because it presents an opportunity.

Beyond health, the Opportunity Gap can be used to explore all kinds of innovations that are riding the exponential curve and making life easier or better. Consider how cryptocurrency allows people to earn and pay for services without a bank. Perhaps you'll draw on an account built by an investment AI system in cyberspace and fund your hyper-extended retirement or your return to school on your 95th birthday. Or one day, a restaurant brand will charge you to send a molecular blueprint over the Internet to your home 3-D printer to "print" a nutritiously custom meal for dinner, perhaps based on a Gordon Ramsay-designed recipe. Maybe a VR company will provide a vacation experience that has the sensory experience of a high-end beach resort in Mexico but fed into a VR experience suit that you wear in an empty warehouse in a strip mall in the suburbs.

These remarkable future technologies remind me of a quote that seems to have originated with sociobiologist Edward O. Wilson and perfectly captures the era we're in. He said, "We have Paleolithic emotions, medieval institutions, and godlike technology."

While this may seem perplexing, it isn't. We will use our god-like technology to upgrade our Stone Age brains and medieval societal structures. We have been doing this for centuries. The only difference today is that we once had more control over what changes to make. Today, however, technology is accelerating, and now *it's driving us*, which will simply force us to adapt faster.

Humans like control and don't always embrace change, so we will feel "disrupted." But we must remember that we are only disrupted if we allow ourselves to feel that way. Embracing it, being open-minded, and adapting to what's coming is a choice. Let's choose to be wowed and inspired.

A Practical Guide to Applying the Opportunity Gap to Your Health

Now, I know there has been a lot of conjecture here and ideas that are exciting to explore but not immediately practical. So, for those of you who are longing for immediate gratification, here are some health tools that are in the Opportunity Gap that you can use today.

Already, millions of people are choosing to bypass their doctor and take control of their health by monitoring their metrics. Wearable devices are certainly helping, and I bet if I could look at your wrist, you might be wearing a smartwatch right now, or you might be considering one. If so, that's good news. Go for it and wear it for a better you.

What you may not know is you have access to numerous affordable, personalized at-home test kits (like the Viome tests). Besides Viome's Full Body Intelligence Test, which provides data on microbiome and cellular health, there are only a few other tests you need to do annually to gather the data points you need to make informed health choices and stay healthy.

There are six tests we recommend that everyone should take. If you selected the most expensive ones and did them annually, they would cost—in total—less than $2500, and they would provide you with the data you need to stay healthy (and keep yourself from spending thousands more as you get older). For a more budget-conscious approach, and depending on your needs and your state of health, you could spend as little as $500 to $1000 per year to stay healthy.

Here is a summary of the tests we recommend. Note that we have provided a more detailed list of all the tests worth exploring on our website, TheYouthFormula.com.

- **Metatranscriptomics microbiome tests**—These are the tests that Viome offers. They provide a comprehensive analysis of genetic material from all organisms in a sample and their functions, interactions, and roles in the human body. They can also reveal which pre-disease states are forming in the body at a molecular level so we can get ahead of them. The Full Body Intelligence Test also includes data on cellular health and considers DNA.[155] **Price Range:** $129–$599

- **Body composition scans**—For low-cost and easy-to-find body scans, look for a DEXA Scan. It measures bone density and body composition. It helps assess risks for osteoporosis and fractures. It can also tell you about body fat and muscle mass. With this test, you can gain insights into how much fat your body has and in what areas.[156] We also recommend the AMRA BCP Scan. It is a more costly body composition scan that uses MRI technology to provide detailed measurements of fat and muscle volumes. It was approved in the U.S. in 2020 and is offered at select MRI centers. **Price Range:** $50 to $100 (DEXA) / $400 to $1000 (AMRA)

- **Toxicity tests**—These include Heavy Metal and Mycotoxin Tests. The Heavy Metal Test measures blood levels of metals like lead and mercury (among others), that may have been introduced through the environment and/or via your diet. Mycotoxin Tests detect harmful mold metabolites that are associated with diseases such as kidney toxicity, immune suppression, and neurotoxicity.[157] **Price Range:** $80–$399

- **Hormone tests**—Hormonal imbalances, detectable through these tests, can surface issues in the body's glands. Hormones play key roles in regulating growth, mood, stress response, metabolism, and sexual functions, among other systems.[158] **Price Range:** $150–$549

- **Food sensitivity tests**—There are a variety of tests on the market that offer insights into what foods may be causing negative symptoms. Viome's tests do not currently profile specific antibody responses to foods, however, we are exploring this.[158] **Price Range:** $99–$300

- **Nutrition metabolite tests**—These tests analyze substances produced by a person's metabolism. They show how well your body is using nutrients.[159] **Price Range:** $259–$679

All these tests, except for the DEXA scan, use an at-home collection kit to collect biological samples, which are sent to a lab.

Anyone who's serious about healthspan should also regularly monitor standard blood biomarkers, such as HbA1C, apoB, and hsCRP. Many labs performed annually, such as HbA1c/lipids, should be done more frequently, every 3-6 months, depending on your health status. And there are many other labs you should have evaluated that are not a part of standard physical labs, such as homocysteine, uric acid, and lp(a), among others.[160] This information may seem a little daunting, but we provide further information on this at TheYouthFormula.com.

While many experts predict the hospital of the future will be our home, we are already seeing an early version of this trend today using these kits.

Millions of people are already taking advantage of these tests (and other affordable health tools like wearable devices and trackers) to achieve better health outcomes, and they will lead to greater rates of life extension for all. Soon, celebrating superagers for reaching their 100th birthday will be commonplace. We'll have to shift to celebrating those that make it to 125 and beyond.

Living With Purpose

In the final pages of this book, here's a little bit of philosophical rocket fuel to get you into action to help you put all the learning from this book into motion. It also comes from my heart because this wisdom has served me well personally, and if there is just one thing to use every day for the rest of your very long life, I hope it is this!

There is a secret hack to my Hierarchy of Longevity: When you focus on the top layer, all the other layers become easier to achieve. This is true of Maslow's hierarchy, too.

Here's an example of how it can play out, Maslow-style:

One morning, you're in line at a coffee shop. You're at a stage in your life where you've achieved the first three areas of the Maslow hierarchy. You have food in the fridge and a nice home to keep you safe and warm (physiological needs, level 1). You have a healthy body and a satisfying job (safety and security needs, level 2). You also have a wonderful family and a good group of friends (love and belonging needs, level 3). So, your main focus in life is career satisfaction (self-esteem needs, so level 4 is so far unmet).

As you stand in line, you feel stressed about your upcoming work day. Then, you hear a student behind you talking to a friend about being broke. You choose at that moment to act with the characteristics of a self-actualized person (level 5). Inspired by memories of your own financial struggles at school, you buy the student a coffee as a nice, seemingly trivial gesture.

Your tiny action makes you feel good. It reaffirms your sense of belonging, security, and safety because you have the ability to buy a drink for a stranger. And so, for the rest of the day, you feel great. You get a burst of energy, and you bring that to work, which fuels your ability to make money, connect with others, and succeed in your role. Taking action related to the top layer is access to personal power and makes the other layers easier to achieve by bringing them into greater focus.

You can use the Hierarchy of Longevity in a similar manner. Focusing on purpose (level 5) is a way to make all the other areas of health a greater focus. When you have a purpose you become more likely to want to stay healthy to be able to pursue it. Purpose makes it easier to make the right choices.

This is true for me. I could never have achieved entrepreneurial success if I wasn't healthy. I want to eat well and stay fit so I can keep pursuing moonshots. I also take actions to de-stress so I can continue to pursue my missions. Sleep is also a priority for me. Those close to me know I am crazy about getting great sleep. I want to feel rested because I'm excited to get up in the morning. Feeling physically good then inspires me to keep pursuing my purpose.

When humans have a purpose, we are remarkable, and, fascinatingly, the Universe comes to our aid. It feels as though we get what we need when we need it.

The purpose-health connection has also been validated by longevity science. Numerous studies confirm that purpose reduces a person's risk of heart disease, stroke, and depression and is also linked to longer lifespans. People with a clear purpose are better at adapting to change and more resilient when facing life challenges. In recent years, here is what longevity scientists have learned about purpose and its role in health:

People with a clear purpose are better at adapting to change and more resilient

- Individuals with a strong sense of purpose have a lower risk of death from all causes compared to those with a lower sense of purpose.[161]
- People with a high sense of purpose have a significantly reduced risk of heart attack among those with coronary artery disease. A heightened sense of purpose correlates to a lower likelihood of experiencing strokes.[162]
- A greater sense of purpose substantially decreases the risk of Alzheimer's disease and cognitive decline in older adults.[163]

- Older adults with a sense of purpose experience better physical function and exhibit a lower risk of weak grip strength and slower walking speeds.[164]
- Purpose is a key part of the lives of superagers, as demonstrated by the famous longevity research by Dan Buettner, who identified the Blue Zones, areas of the world with large populations of centenarians living in Okinawa, Sardinia, Nicoya, Icaria, and Loma Linda.[165]

Purpose also shows up in evolutionary theory. Many conscious evolutionary theorists suggest that when we individually and collectively tap into purpose, we awaken an evolutionary impulse within us that drives positive growth for ourselves and others. According to some experts, the crises and challenges humanity faces are essential catalysts for evolutionary change. They spur our species towards increased unity, innovation, and consciousness.[166]

From this perspective, humanity's current challenges, which some say could lead to a sixth mass extinction, are actually propelling us toward our next evolutionary leap. Through our struggles and learning, we gain insights that help us create better tools to prevent, repair, and heal the world's greatest problems.

We humans are at a crucial turning point. Unlike our ancestors, we now possess the capability to *actively direct our evolution*. If we look back at previous evolutionary stages, they were driven by natural selection. We had no control over our destiny. However, now, with our capacity for higher intellect, augmented by technological tools we have created, we can control the future of humankind. We are at a juncture where the combination of our awareness and technological advancements has made us active participants in our evolutionary journey rather than mere onlookers.[167] How incredible is that?

This is why purpose is part of my ethos. Life is better. There is a magical relationship between purpose and health. When we have a purpose, we are likely to stay youthful. Purpose provides a reason to stay healthy, and as we stay healthy, we keep going.

There is a magical relationship between purpose and health.

So, to prime you for living well and living healthy, I leave you with this question: What can you do to live purposefully? I have found there are two ways. We can:

1. Choose a purpose to pursue
2. Be purposeful at any moment

Let's look at each one.

How to Choose Your Purpose

To figure out your purpose, ask yourself these questions. These are my favorites:

- What do people who know you well say that you're obsessed about? Or what are you so obsessed about that it is as easy and automatic as breathing?
- What major global problem do you struggle with? What problem is desperate for a solution?

- What major crisis in your life did you once not only survive but from which you learned great skills? (It's often linked to your obsession and skills.)

You can also do a simple fill-in-the-blank exercise. Ask yourself "what if" or "imagine" and fill in the blank on what comes next. It goes like this:

Imagine living on a different planet. What would it take for us to survive and to thrive?

What if solving world hunger is less about growing more food and more about why we need food as an energy source at all?

What if climate change wasn't simply about reducing fossil fuels used but really about preventing forest fires, which generate more carbon than fossil fuels?

Now, what audacious goal can you come up with by asking better questions?

Your answer will give you a hint about what you care about. From that you might want to formulate a moonshot that you take on. You could use it to launch a business, create an initiative inside an existing one, or start a movement by bringing like-minded people together.

The second approach to harnessing your purpose is to live purposefully from moment to moment.

Be Purposeful at Every Moment

Living purposefully is an active process. It is a moment-to-moment choice. If we search for it, we can find purpose in everything we do.

Purpose becomes easy to achieve when we expand our perspective to see that the smallest actions have a major impact. With health, this is certainly true. Small actions, in aggregate, can bring great health. For example, there is a purpose in brushing our teeth. Pausing to be present while engaging in this two-minute daily activity keeps our health in check. Making a meal for our family can be a mundane or purposeful act. There is value there. The family needs the meal to be nourished and come together.

So, ask yourself any day, any time: What can I do to bring purpose to this moment? And make it a practice. You will find life gets more fulfilling, and you will have a reason to want to stick around and be healthy.

When I wake up, I think, *Wow, I feel alive and strong!* I look at my wife, Anu, in the morning and take a moment to say, *Thank you, Universe, for this woman.* When I eat, I take a moment to pause and appreciate my food. These small actions matter. I know it's easy to skip them, but they add up, and they shape your attitude. So, pause and appreciate every moment. It is a simple action we can all engage in.

And, if you're ever grasping for purpose, choose your health. It is a great place to start. Why not even practice that now? Bring purpose to these words you're reading on the page.

One Body, One Life

Think about a moment when you were in a blissful state, where your body and mind were totally relaxed. For many people, it's when they are on vacation.

If we take a week off, after a few days of relaxation and with a few more days ahead of us, we often find ourselves with an overwhelming sense of joy and connection with life. With our brains no longer focused on work, taking care of the household, or paying bills, we float along with life as if we're tubing down a stream, though that might actually be the case.

Experts say that when our brain is not focused on tasks, we are no longer in an activity state called Task Mode Network (TMN). Instead, we are in a Default Mode Network (DMN) where creativity flows.[168] We get great ideas when we are relaxed. We feel good. We reconnect with our true nature. We remember what life is about. When we get too caught up with work and we are busy, it's easy to forget. When we are fed, rested, and happy, we are more loving, too. We want to live, experience, and share. We want to connect.

It's interesting that when most of us experience this on vacation, we are in a moment when we hit all the levels of the Hierarchy of Longevity. We are well-fed and well-rested. We generally have more time to engage in fitness activities, even if it's simply a walk to breakfast or a hike to the top of a hill to take in a view.

This is the reason health matters. We want to invoke this state perpetually, not just on vacation a few times a year. We want it as much as possible. But we truly must choose it.

And so, I hope you have found something wondrous for yourself in this book. Perhaps you see your life differently now. Perhaps you see what is possible for your health in a new way. Perhaps you see new actions to take. Do the work. Find your purpose. And be sure to create a personal health moonshot.

Here is mine: To live longer than Dadi and experience every moment of my life with great health and energy so I have the body and the mind to keep pursuing moonshots and live a very long and purposeful life.

With that, I am turning it over to you. It is your turn to ask the questions. To imagine what is possible.

- What do you wish for?
- What do you want for your health?
- What do you want for your life?

We all get one body, and what we do with it matters. And now, finally, we have the most incredible technological tools to understand and treat it better. To make that happen, you must believe it. You must declare a healthy life for yourself. You must commit.

So, eat what your body needs, move it well, and seek rejuvenation by resting it well. Do more of what brings you joy. A lot of that comes from your purpose. Find your obsession, make it a moonshot, and pursue it with every cell of your being.

Let's ensure our bodies are well and vibrant and primed for greatness because without a healthy body, we can't do anything meaningful in this lifetime. Make this one life count.

The Mindset Shift

If you take one insight from this chapter, let it be this...

If you want to live a long, healthy disease-free life, there are personalized health tools that make it possible and simpler. Overtime, they will get more sophisticated. To take advantage of them, you must stay informed and use them when they become available.

One principle makes health simpler: live with purpose.

Key Insights

- We have never experienced a time of more technological growth and convergence, and it's led to more opportunities for each and every individual.
- Technology will continue to accelerate. We will adapt societal structures to keep up. We will use more tools to upgrade our biology.
- The Opportunity Gap is a principle that demonstrates the difference in growth between science and technology and institutions and government.
- As a result of The Opportunity Gap, individuals have more control over their lives and personal power than in previous generations.
- The trend of rapidly accelerating technology and science is shaping healthcare, and it will lead to

the era of precision medicine, where health will become more and more personalized. First generation precision medicine tools are already available from companies like Viome.

- To take advantage of the best tools for health, we must keep an eye on trends and monitor technology and health news.
- Useful tests to gain data on your body are: Body scans like DEXA scan, toxicity tests, food sensitivity tests, nutrition metabolite tests, hormone tests, and tests for a complete genetic picture, which Viome offers.
- Once we know our body's data and have a scientific understanding of each critical area of health—nutrition, stress, fitness, sleep, mindset—then we can use that information to make the best choices.
- Health starts and ends with purpose. We must choose to have a healthy body and believe we can. The right mindset will have us take the right actions.
- The way we think may be one of the most important skills for a great body and life.
- Living with purpose is a way to keep health a focus because when we have a mission, we need to stay healthy to achieve it.
- There are two ways to live purposefully: 1) pursue a moonshot, and 2) be purposeful.
- Pursuing a moonshot requires deep thought. Ask yourself the three questions: *Why this? Why now? Why me?* to figure it out.
- Being purposeful is a moment-to-moment choice you can make.
- We have one body and one life. Without our body, we can't do much, so we must take care of it.

AFTERWORD

The primary goal of this book is awareness. Our objective is to empower readers like you to pursue the goal of lifelong health. In this book, you learned about our work and research at Viome. If you're inspired to learn more and start your journey of precision nutrition, visit Viome.com.

If you enjoyed this book, please share what you've learned. We need more people in this world to take control of their health and feel empowered. For more information on resources used in this book, to learn more about health coaching certification programs, and to browse our collections of research by disease, visit TheYouthFormula.com.

END NOTES

Chapter 1

1. "Obesity and Overweight," *World Health Organization*, last accessed January 2024, https://www.who.int/news-room/fact-sheets/detail/obesity-and-overweight.

2. "Noncommunicable Diseases," *World Health Organization*, last accessed January 2024, https://www.who.int/news-room/fact-sheets/detail/noncommunicable-diseases.

3. Institute of Medicine (US) Committee for the Study of the Future of Public Health, "A History of the Public Health System," *National Academies Press US*. (1988) https://www.ncbi.nlm.nih.gov/books/NBK218224.

4. University of Alberta, "Your DNA is Not Your Destiny -- Or a Good Predictor of Your Health," *Science Daily*, last accessed January 2024, https://www.sciencedaily.com/releases/2019/12/191219142739.htm

5. Maria Jackson, Leah Marks, Gerhard H.W. May, "The Genetic Basis for Disease," *Essays Biochem.* 62(5): 643–723. (December 2018): https://doi.org/10.1042/EBC20170053.

6. Linda Geddes, "How Your Body Processes Food is Only Partially Down to Your Genes." *NewScientist*, June 2019.

7. Tanecia Mitchell et al, "Dietary Oxalate and Kidney Stone Formation," *Am J Physiol Renal Physiol.* 316(3), (March 2019): F409–F413, https://doi.org/ 10.1152/ajprenal.00373.2018.

8. Facts & Factors, "Weight Loss and Weight Management Market Size," last accessed January 2024, http://latest-global-weight-loss-and-weight-management.pdf.

9. LeWine, Howard E., "Taking Aim At Belly Fat." *Harvard Health Publishing*, last accessed March 26, 2024, https://www.health.harvard.edu/newsletter_article/taking-aim-at-belly-fat.

10. Aaiza Tahreem et al., "Fad Diets: Facts and Fiction." *Frontiers in Nutrition*, 9, (July 2022): 960922, https://doi.org/10.3389/fnut.2022.960922.

11. Yegor E. Yegorov et al., "The Link Between Chronic Stress and Accelerated Aging." *Biomedicines*,

8(7), (July 2020): 198, https://doi.org/10.3390/biomedicines8070198.

12. Ron Sender, Shai Fuchs, and Ron Milo, "Revised Estimates for the Number of Human and Bacteria Cells in the Body" *PLOS Biol.* 14(8), (August 2016): e1002533, https://doi.org/10.1371/journal.pbio.1002533.

13. Haseeb Anwar et al., "Gut Microbiome: A New Organ System in the Body." *Parasitology and Microbiology Research*, (November 2019): https://doi.org/10.5772/intechopen.89634.

14. "Dirt Poor: Have Fruits and Vegetables Become Less Nutritious?" *Scientific America*, April 27, 2011. https://www.scientificamerican.com/article/soil-depletion-and-nutrition-loss.

Chapter 2

15. "A History of How Humans Learned to Fly," *Let's Talk Science*, last modified December 15, 2021, https://letstalkscience.ca/educational-resources/backgrounders/a-history-how-humans-learned-fly.

16. "Fia World Land Speed Records," *FIA World Records*, last accessed December 2023, https://www.fia.com/fia-world-land-speed-records.

17. "A Speedy Look at Speed," *Milwaukee Public Museum*, last accessed February 2024, https://mpm.edu/plan-visit/theater-planetarium/starry-messenger/planetarium-newsletter-september-2021.

18. "Four-Minute Mile," Wikipedia, last accessed January 2024, https://en.wikipedia.org/wiki/Four-minute_mile.

19. "Ending Health Care's Affordability Crisis Begins With Actions to Fix State Markets," Route-Fifty, last modified February 27, 2024, https://www.route-fifty.com/finance/2024/02/ending-health-cares-affordability-crisis-begins-actions-fix-state-markets/394484.

20. Pifer, Rebecca, "US Health Spending to Surpass $7T by 2031, CMS Actuaries Say," *Healthcare Dive*, last modified June 15, 2023, https://www.healthcaredive.com/news/us-health-spending-projections-cms-covid-ira.

21. The Commonwealth Fund, "U.S Health Care from a Global Perspective, 2022: Accelerating Spending, Worsening Outcomes," last modified January 31, 2023, https://www.commonwealthfund.org/publications/issue-briefs/2023/jan/us-health-care-global-perspective-2022.

22. The Commonwealth Fund, "U.S Health Care from a Global Perspective, 2022: Accelerating Spending, Worsening Outcomes," last modified January 31, 2023, https://www.commonwealthfund.org/publications/issue-briefs/2023/jan/us-health-care-global-perspective-2022.

23. "Debunking Myths About Being Fat," *Science Friday*, last modified May 19, 2023, https://www.sciencefriday.com/segments/debunking-myths-fat-research-book.

24. The Commonwealth Fund, "U.S Health Care from a Global Perspective, 2022: Accelerating

Spending, Worsening Outcomes," last modified January 31, 2023, https://www.commonwealth-fund.org/publications/issue-briefs/2023/jan/us-health-care-global-perspective-2022.

25. Bill Gross, "The Single Biggest Reason Why Startups Succeed," filmed March 2015 at TED Conference, video, https://www.ted.com/talks/bill_gross_the_single_biggest_reason_why_start_ups_succeed.

26. Bill Gross, "The Single Biggest Reason Why Startups Succeed," filmed March 2015 at TED Conference, video, https://www.ted.com/talks/bill_gross_the_single_biggest_reason_why_start_ups_succeed.

27. Bill Gross, "The Single Biggest Reason Why Startups Succeed," filmed March 2015 at TED Conference, video, https://www.ted.com/talks/bill_gross_the_single_biggest_reason_why_start_ups_succeed.

28. National Human Genome Research Institute, "The Coast of Sequencing a Human Genome," last accessed January 2024, https://www.genome.gov/about-genomics/fact-sheets/Sequencing-Human-Genome-cost.

29. "History of Personal Computers," Wikipedia, last accessed February 2024, https://en.wikipedia.org/wiki/History_of_personal_computers.

30. "Moore's Law," Wikipedia, last accessed February 2024, https://en.wikipedia.org/wiki/Moore%27s_law.

31. "Your Brain is Wired for Linear Thinking. Learn Exponential Thinking Instead," *Big Think*, last modified December 19, 2019, https://bigthink.com/

plus/your-brain-is-wired-for-linear-thinking-learn-exponential-thinking-instead.

32. Antonio Regalado, "More Than 26 Million People Have taken an At Home Ancestry Test," *MIT Technology Review*, February 11, 2019, https://www.technologyreview.com/2019/02/11/103446/more-than-26-million-people-have-taken-an-at-home-ancestry-test.

33. Own, "Short: The DNA Journey," video, last accessed December 2023, https://www.youtube.com/watch?v=secwZOPS074.

34. Institute of Medicine (US) Committee on Assessing Interactions Among Social, Behavioral, and Genetic Factors in Health, *Genetics and Health. Genes, Behavior, and the Social Environment: Moving Beyond the Nature/Nurture Debate*, National Academies Press US, (2006): https://www.ncbi.nlm.nih.gov/books/NBK19932.

35. "The Human Genome Project," National Human Genome Research, last accessed January 2024, https://www.genome.gov/human-genome-project.

36. Francis S. Collins, M.D., Ph.D. and Leslie Fink, "The Human Genome Project," Alcohol Health and Research World, 19(3), (1995): 190–195, https://www.ncbi.nlm.nih.gov/pmc/articles/PMC6875757.

37. Wade, Nicholas. "Experts Say They Have Key to Rice Genes." *New York Times,* April 2002, https://www.nytimes.com/2002/04/05/us/experts-say-they-have-key-to-rice-genes.html.

38. Ankit Gupta, Rasna Gupta, and Ram Lakhan Singh, "Microbes and Environment," *Principles and Applications of Environmental Biotechnology for a Sustainable Future*. 43–84. (October 2016): https://doi.org/10.1007/978-981-10-1866-4_3.

39. Science in the News, "The 99 Percent…of The Human Genome," *Harvard Kenneth C. Griffin Graduate School of Arts and Sciences*, October 1, 2012, https://sitn.hms.harvard.edu/flash/2012/issue127a.

40. Leaf, Clifton. "What Elephants Can Teach Us About Alzheimer's Disease" *Fortune*. August 3, 2018, https://fortune.com/2018/08/03/alzheimers-elephants-memory.

41. "Ribonucleic Acid, RNA," National Human Genome Research Institute, last modified June 30, 2024, https://www.genome.gov/genetics-glossary/RNA-Ribonucleic-Acid.

Chapter 3

42. "Airbus A380," Wikipedia, last accessed Feb 2024, https://en.wikipedia.org/wiki/Airbus_A380.

43. Jacobo Prisco, "20 Astonishing Facts About the A380 Superjumbo," *CNN*, December 18, 2021, https://www.cnn.com/travel/article/airbus-a380-superjumbo-astonishing-facts/index.html.

44. "Airbus A380," Wikipedia, last accessed Feb 2024, https://en.wikipedia.org/wiki/Airbus_A380.

45. Systems Biology, "Systems Biology: A Short Overview," last accessed February 2024, https://youtube.com/watch?v=vWSsNi5uFVY

46. Systems Biology, "Systems Biology: A Short Overview," last accessed February 2024, https://youtube.com/watch?v=vWSsNi5uFVY.

47. Systems Biology, "Systems Biology: A Short Overview," last accessed February 2024, https://youtube.com/watch?v=vWSsNi5uFVY.

48. "Quadrillion," Googology Wiki, last accessed March 2024, https://googology.fandom.com/wiki/Quadrillion.

49. "Early Life on Earth—Animal Origins." Smithsonian, last accessed February 2024, https://naturalhistory.si.edu/education/teaching-resources/life-science/early-life-earth-animal-origins.

50. Carina M. Schlebusch et al., "Southern African Ancient Genomes Estimate Modern Human Divergence to 350,000 to 260,000 years ago," *Science*. Vol. 358, Issue 6363, (September 2017): 652-655, https://doi.org/10.1126/science.aao6266.

51 Carina M. Schlebusch et al., "Southern African Ancient Genomes Estimate Modern Human Divergence to 350,000 to 260,000 years ago," *Science*. Vol. 358, Issue 6363, (September 2017): 652-655, https://doi.org/10.1126/science.aao6266.

52. Greshko, Michael., "How Many Cells Are in the Human Body," *National Geographic*, last accessed February 2024, https://www.nationalgeographic.com/science/article/160111-microbiome-estimate-count-ratio-human-health-science.

53. The American Society for Microbiology, "The Microbial World: Foundation of the Biosphere,"

The American Society for Microbiology, Washington, DC, (1997): ncbi.nlm.nih.gov/books/NBK562919.

54. Nick Lane, "The Unseen World: Reflections of Leeuwenbauk," *The Royal Society Publishing Philosophical Transactions,* B.370 (1666), (April 2015): 20140344, https://doi.org/10.1098/rstb.2014.0344.

55. "Germ Theory," Britannica, last modified May 22, 2024, https://www.britannica.com/science/germ-theory.

56. Jack Gilbert et al., "Current Understanding of the Human Microbiome," *Nature Medicine.* 24 (4), (April 2018): 392-400, https://doi.org/10.1038/nm.4517.

57. Jane Nysten, "Can We Microbe-Manage Our Vitamin Acquisition for Better Health?" *PLOS Pathogens,* 19(5), (May 2023): e1011361, https://doi.org/10.1371/journal.ppat.1011361.

58. American Society for Microbiology. *FAQ: Human Microbiome,* (American Society for Microbiology, 2013), https://www.ncbi.nlm.nih.gov/books/NBK562894.

59. Cristina Kalbermatter et al. "Maternal Microbiota, Early Life Colonization and Breast Milk Drive Immune Development in the Newborn." *Frontiers in Immunology,* 12: 683022. (May 2021): https://doi.org/10.3389/fimmu.2021.683022.

60. Hongyan Chen and Dingliang Tan, "Cesarean Section or Natural Childbirth? Cesarean Birth May Damage Your Health." *Frontiers in Psychology,* 10: 351. (February 2019): https://doi.org/10.3389/fpsyg.2019.00351.

61. Frontiers in Systems Biology, "A Complete Guide to Human Microbiomes: Body Niches, Transmission, Development, Dysbiosis, and Restoration," *Frontiers in Systems Biology*, Vol. 2 (July 2022): https://doi.org/10.3389/fsysb.2022.951403.

62. Frontiers in Systems Biology, "A Complete Guide to Human Microbiomes: Body Niches, Transmission, Development, Dysbiosis, and Restoration," *Frontiers in Systems Biology*, Vol. 2 (July 2022): https://doi.org/10.3389/fsysb.2022.951403.

63. K Krishnan, T Chen, and BJ Paster, "A Practical Guide to the Oral Microbiome and its Relation to Health and Disease," *Oral Diseases*. 23(3), (April 2017): 276–286, https://doi.org/10.1111/odi.12509.

64. Frontiers in Systems Biology. "A Complete Guide to Human Microbiomes: Body Niches, Transmission, Development, Dysbiosis, and Restoration," *Frontiers in Systems Biology*, Vol. 2 (July 2022): https://doi.org/10.3389/fsysb.2022.951403.

65. "Types of Microorganisms," Britannica, last accessed January 2024, https://www.britannica.com/science/microbiology/Types-of-microorganisms.

66. Arianna K. DeGruttola. "Current Understanding of Dysbiosis Disease in Human and Animal Models," *Inflammatory Bowel Diseases*. 22, 5, (May 2016): 1137–1150, https://doi.org/10.1097/MIB.0000000000000750.

67. "Antimicrobial Resistance," World Health Organization, last modified November 2023, https://www.who.int/news-room/fact-sheets/detail/antimicrobial-resistance.

68. "What is Antimicrobial Resistance and How Can We Tackle It?" World Economic Forum, last modified November 2023, https://www.weforum.org/agenda/2023/11/antimicrobial-resistance-superbugs-antibiotics.

69. Microbe Media. "Invisible Extinction," Directed by Steve Lawrence and Sarah Schenck. (2022; United States) Netflix.

70. "Stop Using Antiobiotics in Healthy Animals to Prevent the Spread of Antibiotic Resistance," World Health Organization, last accessed November 2023, https://www.who.int/news/item/07-11-2017-stop-using-antibiotics-in-healthy-animals-to-prevent-the-spread-of-antibiotic-resistance.

71. Michael Worobey et al., "The Huanan Seafood Wholesale Market in Wuhan Was the Early Epicenter of the Covid-19 Pandemic," *Science*, Vol. 377 (6609), (July 2022): 951-959, https:///doi.org/10.1126/science.abp8715.

72. Muyesaier Tudi et al., "Agriculture Development, Pesticide Application and Its Impact on the Environment," *International Journal of Environmental Research and Public Health*, 18,3, (February 2021): 1112, https:///doi.org/10.3390/ijerph18031112.

73. Stacy Colino. "Fruits and Vegetables are Less Nutritious Than They Used to Be," *National Geographic*, last modified, August 2022, https://www.nationalgeographic.com/magazine/article/fruits-and-vegetables-are-less-nutritious-than-they-used-to-be.

74. "Dirt Poor: Have Fruits and Vegetables Become Less Nutritious?" *Scientific American*, last accessed February 2024, https://www.scientificamerican.com/article/soil-depletion-and-nutrition-loss.

75. "Processed Foods and Health," *The Nutrition Source, Harvard T.H. Chan School of Public Health*, last accessed February 2024, https://www.hsph.harvard.edu/nutritionsource/processed-foods.

76. "Cancer: Carcinogenicity of the Consumption of Red Meat and Processed Meat," The World Health Organizations, last modified October 2025, https://www.who.int/news-room/questions-and-answers/item/cancer-carcinogenicity-of-the-consumption-of-red-meat-and-processed-meat.

77. Graham Lawton, "The Shocking Decline of Earth's Microbiome," *New Scientist*, April 12, 2023, https://www.newscientist.com/article/mg25834344-900-the-shocking-decline-of-earths-microbiome-and-how-to-save-it.

78. Graham Lawton, "The Shocking Decline of Earth's Microbiome," *New Scientist*, April 12, 2023, https://www.newscientist.com/article/mg25834344-900-the-shocking-decline-of-earths-microbiome-and-how-to-save-it.

79. Magellan Studio, "The Gut: Our Second Brain," Directed by Cecile Denjean. (2012).

80. Sharon Terlep, "Hand Sanitizer Sales Jumped 600 in 2020," *The Wall Street Journal*, January 22, 2021, https://www.wsj.com/articles/hand-sanitizer-

sales-jumped-600-in-2020-purell-maker-bets-against-a-post-pandemic-collapse-11611311430.

81. McHugh, Jess. "How the 1918 Pandemic Changed America," *The Washington Post*. November 13, 2022. https://www.washingtonpost.com/history/2022/11/13/1918-flu-pandemic-women-science.

82. Pamela DenBesten and Wu Li, "Chronic Fluoride Toxicity: Dental Fluorosis," Monographs in Oral Science, *Monographs in Oral Science,* 22, (June 2011): 81-96, https:///doi.org/10.1159/000327028.

83. Joanna A. Ruszkiewicz et al. "Neurotoxic Effect of Active Ingredients in Sunscreen Products, A Contemporary Review," *Toxicology Reports*, 4, (May 2017): 245-259, https:///doi.org/10.1016/j.toxrep.2017.05.006.

84. "What is Homeostasis?" *Scientific American*, last accessed January 2024, https://www.scientificamerican.com/article/what-is-homeostasis. https:///doi.org/10.1159/000327028.

Chapter 4

85. "You Are Your Brain," *Healthy Brains, Cleveland Clinic*, last accessed February 2024, https://healthybrains.org/brain-facts.

86. Vanessa Aguiar-Pulido et al., "Metagenomics, Metatranscriptomics, and Metabolomics Approaches for Microbiome Analysis," *Evolutionary Bioinformatics*, Vol. 12, supply 1, (May 2016): 5-16, https:///doi.org/10.4137/EBO.S36436.

87. Vanessa Aguiar-Pulido et al., "Metagenomics, Metatranscriptomics, and Metabolomics Approaches for Microbiome Analysis," *Evolutionary Bioinformatics*, Vol. 12, supply 1, (May 2016): 5-16, https:///doi.org/10.4137/EBO.S36436.

88. Nojoud Al Fayez et al., "Recent Advancement in mRNA Vaccine Development and Application," *Pharmaceutics*, 15, 7 (July 2023): 1972, https:///doi.org/10.3390/pharmaceutics15071972.

89. Gregory Hardy, "Big Data Health Science Center Brings Big Minds, Big Ideas," *University of South Carolina*, last modified April 22, 2024, https://www.sc.edu/uofsc/posts/2024/04/big-data-health-science-center-big-ideas.php.

90. "When You're Stuck in the Sand," Bedtime Math, last accessed March 2024, https://bedtimemath.org/fun-math-buried-in-sand.

91. Jeremy Appleton, "The Gut-Brain Axis: Influence of Microbiota on Mood and Mental Health," *Integrative Medicine (Encinitas)*, 17, 4 (August 2018): 28-32, https://www.ncbi.nlm.nih.gov/pmc/articles/PMC6469458.

92. Magellan Studio. "The Gut: Our Second Brain," Directed by Cecile Denjean. (2012).

93. Magellan Studio. "The Gut: Our Second Brain," Directed by Cecile Denjean. (2012).

94. Caitriona M. Guinane and Paul D. Cotter, "Role of the Gut Microbiota in Health and Chronic Gastrointestinal Disease: Understanding a Hidden Metabolic Organ," *Therapeutic Advances in*

Gastroenterology, 6, 4: (July 2013): 295–308, https:///
doi.org/ 10.1177/1756283X1348299.

95. Erin Ferranti et al, "20 Things You Didn't Know
About the Human Gut Microbiome," *Journal
of Cardiovascular Nursing*, 29, 6 (December
2014): 479-481, https:///doi.org/ 10.1097/
JCN.0000000000000166.

96. Vincent Ho, "Your Poo is (Mostly) Alive, Here's What's
In It," *The Conversation*, October 31, 2018, https://
theconversation.com/your-poo-is-mostly-alive-here
s-whats-in-it-102848.

97. Ana Sandoiu, "Nutrition: Even Identical Twins
Respond Differently to Foods," *MedicalNews Today*,
June 20, 2019, https://www.medicalnewstoday.com/
articles/325521.

98. Steven Brown, "Can What You Eat Give You
Kidney Stones?" *WebMD*, March 14, 2024.
https://www.webmd.com/kidney-stones/kidney-
stones-food-causes.

99. Ya-Jie Xiao, Miao Hu, and Brian Tomlinson, "Effects
of Grapefruit Juice on Cortisol Metabolism in
Healthy Male Chinese Subjects," Food and Chemical
Toxicology, Vol. 74, (December 2014): 85-90, https://
doi.org/10.1016/j.fct.2014.09.012.

100. "Turmeric," *MountSinai,* last accessed March 2024,
https://www.mountsinai.org/health-library/herb/
turmeric.

101. D. B. Nandini et al., "Sulforaphane in Broccoli:
The Green Chemoprevention!! Role in Cancer
Prevention and Therapy," Journal of Oral and

Maxillofacial Pathology, 24, 2, (August 2020): 405, https://doi.org/10.4103/jomfp.JOMFP_126_19.

102. William R. Lovallo et al., "Caffeine Stimulation of Cortisol Secretion Across the Waking Hours in Relation to Caffeine Intake Levels," *Psychosomatic Medicine*, 67, 5 (2005): 734–739, https://doi.org/10.1097/01.psy.0000181270.20036.06.

103. Dawit T Zemedikun et al., "Burden of Chronic Diseases Associated with Periodontal Diseases: a Retrospective Cohort Study Using UK Primary Care Data," *BMJ Open*, 11, 12 (December 2021): e048296, https://doi.org/10.1136/bmjopen-2020-048296.

104. Monika Singh et al, "Prevalence of Periodontal Disease in Type 2 Diabetes Mellitus Patients: A Cross-sectional Study," *Contemporary Clinical Dentistry*, 10, 2, (June 2019): 349–357, https://doi.org/10.4103/ccd.ccd_652_18.

105. Mihir S. Kulkarni et al. "Poor Oral Health Linked with Higher Risk of Alzheimer's Disease," *Brain Science*, 13, 11 (November 2023): 1555, https://doi.org/10.3390/brainsci13111555.

106. "Oral Health Problems May Raise Cancer Risk," Harvard, last accessed May 2024, https://www.health.harvard.edu/cancer/oral-health-problems-may-raise-cancer-risk.

107. Shah Saif Jahan et al, "Oral Healthcare during Pregnancy: Its Importance and Challenges in Lower-Middle-Income Countries (LMICs)," *International Journal of Environmental Research*

and Public Health, 19, 17, (September 2022): 10681, https://doi.org/10.3390/ijerph191710681.

108. Masood A. Shammas, "Telomeres, Lifestyle, Cancer, and Aging," *Current Opinion in Clinical Nutrition & Metabolic Care*, 14, 1 (January 2011): 28-34, https://doir.org/10.1097/MCO.0b013e32834121b1.

109. "What Does UI Mean on Vitamin Labels," *Uscriptives*, August 27, 2021, https://uscriptives.com/blogs/what-does-iu-mean-on-vitamin-labels.

110. Santiago Espinosa-Salas and Mauricio Gonzalez-Arias, "Nutrition: Micronutrient Intake, Imbalances, and Interventions," *StatPearls*, last modified September 21, 2023, https://www.ncbi.nlm.nih.gov/books/NBK597352.

111. Julia Niño-Narvión et al, "NAD+ Precursors and Intestinal Inflammation: Therapeutic Insights Involving Gut Microbiota," *Nutrients*, 15, 13, (July 2023): 2992, https://doi.org/10.3390/nu15132992.

112. Manuel H. Janeiro et al. "Implication of Trimethylamine N-Oxide (TMAO) in Disease: Potential Biomarker or New Therapeutic Target," *Nutrients*, 10,10(October 2018):1389, https://doi.org/10.3390/nu10101398.

113. Andressa Louzada Frauche Fernandes et al. Dietary Intake of Tyrosine and Phenylalanine, and P-Cresyl Sulfate Plasma Levels in Non-Dialyzed Patients with Chronic Kidney Disease," *Journal of Nephrology*, 42, 3 (September 2023): 307-314: https://doi.org/10.1590/2175-8239-JBN-2018-0214.

114 "Daily Value on the Nutrition and Supplements Facts Labels," *U.S. Food and Drug Administration*, last accessed June 2024, https://www.fda.gov/food/nutrition-facts-label/daily-value-nutrition-and-supplement-facts-labels.

115. "Bad Breath," *Mayo Clinic*, last accessed March 2024, https://www.mayoclinic.org/diseases-conditions/bad-breath/symptoms-causes.

116. "Sensitivity and Specificity," Wikipedia, last accessed June 2024, https://en.wikipedia.org/wiki/Sensitivity_and_specificity.

117. "What is the Vaginal Microbiome?" *Evvy*, last accessed March 2024, https://evvy.com/blog/vaginal-microbiome.

Chapter 5

118. Saul Mcleod, "Maslow's Hierarchy of Needs," *Simple Psychology*, last modified January 2024, https://www.simplypsychology.org/maslow.html.

119. Saul Mcleod, "Maslow's Hierarchy of Needs," *Simple Psychology*, last modified January 2024, https://www.simplypsychology.org/maslow.html.

120. Habib Yaribeygi et al., "The Impact of Stress on Body Function: A Review," *EXCLI Journal*, 16, (July 2017): 1057–1072, https://doi.org/10.17179/excli2017-480.

121. Tomohiko Kamo et al. "The Impact of Malnutrition on Efficacy of Resistance Training in Community-Dwelling Older Adults," *Physiotherapy*

Research International, (October 2018) https://doi.
org/10.1002/pri.1755.

122. Jay Summer, "Nutrition and Sleep: Diet's Effects
on Sleep," last modified May 10, 2024, https://
www.sleepfoundation.org/nutrition.

123. "Stress Effects on the Body," *American Psychological
Associations,* last modified March 8, 2023, https://
www.apa.org/topics/stress/body.

124. "Stress Effects on the Body," *American Psychological
Associations,* last modified March 8, 2023, https://
www.apa.org/topics/stress/body.

125. "Stress Effects on the Body," *American Psychological
Associations,* last modified March 8, 2023, https://
www.apa.org/topics/stress/body.

126. "Stress Symptoms: Effects on Your Body and
Behavior," *Mayo Clinic,* last accessed February 2024,
https://www.mayoclinic.org/healthy-lifestyle/
stress-management/in-depth/stress-symptoms/
art-20050987.

127. Lela Moore, "How Meditation Changes
the Brain, *PsychCentral,*" last modified June
3, 2021, https://psychcentral.com/blog/
how-meditation-changes-the-brain.

128. "Benefits of Physical Activity," *CDC,* last accessed
June 2024, https://www.cdc.gov/physical-activity-
basics/benefits.

129. "How Can Strength Training Build Healthier
Bodies As We Age?," *National Institute on Aging,* last
modified June 30, 2022, https://www.nia.nih.gov/

news/how-can-strength-training-build-healthie
r-bodies-we-age.

130. Shereen Lehman, "Broken Bones Tied to Increased
Risk of Death for Up to 10 Years," *Reuters*, last
modified August 9, 2018, https://www.reuters.
com/article/idUSKBN1KU2BB.

131. Jennifer Leavitt, "How Much Deep, Light and
REM Sleep Do You Need?" Healthline, last modified January 18, 2024, https://www.healthline.
com/health/how-much-deep-sleep-do-you-need.

132. Nikola Chung et al. "Does the Proximity of Meals
to Bedtime Influence the Sleep of Young Adults?
A Cross Sectional Survey of University Students,"
*International Journal of Environmental Research and
Public Health*, 17, 8 (April 2020): 2677 https://doi.
org/10.3390/ijerph17082677.

133. Eric S. Kim et al. "Sense of Purpose in Life
and Subsequent Physical, Behavioral, and
Psychosocial Health: An Outcome-Wide
Approach," *American Journal of Health Promotion*,
36, 1 (January 2022): 137-147, https://doi.
org/10.1177/08901171211038545.

134. Rosean Bishop, "Does Purpose Play a Positive
Role in Mental Health?" *Mayo Clinic*, last modified
March 15, 2023, https://www.mayoclinichealthsys-
tem.org/hometown-health/speaking-of-health/
purpose-and-mental-health.

135. Dr. Susan Biali, "Cultivate Purpose to Protect
Against Burnout and Improve Well-Being," last

modified March 2023, https://susanbiali.com/ cultivate-purpose-protect-burnout-well-being.

136. "The Neuroscience of Goal-Setting and Its Impacts on Your Culture," *Culture Partner,* last modified September 2022, https://culturepartners.com/ insights/the-neuroscience-of-goal-setting-an d-its-impact-on-your-culture.

137. Kelly Bilodeau, "Will a Purpose Driven Life Help You Live Longer?" last modified November 2019, https://health.harvard.edu/blog/will-a-purpose-driven-life-hel p-you-live-longer-2019112818378.

138. Jenna Fletcher, "What Are the Six Essential Nutrients?" *MedicalNewsToday,* last modified August 2019, https://www.medicalnewstoday. com/articles/326132.

139. "Here's What Food Guides Around the World Look Like," *CBC News,* last modified January 2019, https://www.cbc.ca/news/health/ canada-food-guide-international-guidelines-1 .4962611.

140. "Here's What Food Guides Around the World Look Like," *CBC News,* last modified January 2019, https://www.cbc.ca/news/health/ canada-food-guide-international-guidelines -1.4962611.

141. "Stress Management," *Sing Health,* last accessed June 2024, https://www.singhealth.com.sg/patient-care/ conditions-treatments/stress-management.

142. Stress Management," *Sing Health,* last accessed June 2024, https://www.singhealth.com.sg/patient-care/conditions-treatments/stress-management.

143. "Resilience Training," *Mayo Clinic,* last accessed June 2024, https://www.mayoclinic.org/tests-procedures/resilience-training/about/pac-20394943.

144. Lionel Noah et al. "Effect of Magnesium and Vitamin B6 Supplementation on Mental Health and Quality of Life in Stressed Healthy Adults: Post-hoc Analysis of a Randomised Controlled Trial," *Stress Health,* 37, 5 (December 2021): 1000-1009, https://doi.org/10.1002/smi.3051.

145. Regan Olsson, "Can Certain Foods Increase Stress and Anxiety?" *Banner Health,* last accessed June 2024, https://bannerhealth.com/healthcare blog/better-me/can-certain-foods-increase-stress-and-anxiety.

146. Helen Massy, "Can Certain Foods Boost Your Mood?" last modified March 18, 2024, https://zoe.com/learn/good-mood-food.

147. "Stress Effects on the Body," *American Psychological Associations,* last modified March 8, 2023, https://www.apa.org/topics/stress/body.

148 "Heart-Rate Variability: How it Might Indicate Well-Being," *Harvard Health Publishing,* last modified April 3, 2024, https://www.health.harvard.edu/blog/heart-rate-variability-new-way-track-well-2017112212789.

149. "Exercise & Fitness," *Harvard Health Publishing*, last accessed June 2024, https://www.health.harvard.edu/topics/exercise-and-fitness.

150. Aakash K. Patel et al, "Physiology, Sleep Stages," *StatPearl Publishing* (June 2024): ncbi.nlm.nih.gov/books/NBK526132.

151. "Sleep Tips: 6 Steps to Better Sleep," *Mayo Clinic*, last accessed June 2024, https://www.mayoclinic.org/healthy-lifestyle/adult-health/in-depth/sleep/art-20048379.

Chapter 6

151. "We Need to Talk About a Gap Between Technology and Institutions, Says Entrepreneur," *World Economic Forum*, last accessed June 2024, https://www.weforum.org/videos/gap-between-technology-institutions.

152. "History of Magnetic Resonance Imaging," *Wikipedia*, https://en.wikipedia.org/wiki/History_of_magnetic_resonance_imaging.

153. "Globalization 3.0 Has Shrunk the World," *Yale University*, last accessed June 2024, https://archive-yaleglobal.yale.edu/content/globalization-30-has-shrunk-world.

154. Wei Zhi et al, "Methods for Understanding Microbial Community Structures and Functions in Microbial Fuel Cells: A Review," *Bioresource Technology*, (2014): https://www.sciencedirect.com/science/article/abs/pii/S0960852414012127.

155. Stephanie Booth, "What is a DEXA Scan?" *WebMD*, December 17, 2023, https://www.webmd.com/osteoporosis/dexa-scan.

156. "Body Composition Profile Magnetic Resonances Imaging," *Mayfair Diagnostics*, last accessed June 2024, https://www.radiology.ca/exam/body-composition-profile-magnetic-resonance-imaging.

157. "Heavy Metal Test," *Cleveland Clinic*, last accessed June 2024, https://my.clevelandclinic.org/health/diagnostics/22797-heavy-metal-test.

157. "Understanding Different Types of Hormones Tests," *BodyLogicMD*, https://www.bodylogicmd.com/hormone-testing/hormone-tests.

159. "Third Party Research, Food Sensitivity," last accessed March 2024, https://www.everlywell.com/blog/news-and-info/third-party-research.

160. "Best At-Home Metabolism Tests in 2024," *Healthline*, last accessed June 2024, https://www.healthline.com/health/metabolism-test.

161. Lizzie Lynch, "Longevity Blood Testing: 8 Biomarkers to Check," *Medichecks*, January 2, 2024, https://www.medichecks.com/blogs/longevity/longevity-blood-testing-8-biomarkers-to-check.

162. "Sense of Purpose in Life Linked to Lower Mortality and Cardiovascular Risk," *Wolters Kluwer Health: Lippincott Williams and Wilkins*, Science Daily, last accessed June 2024, https://www.sciencedaily.com/releases/2015/12/151203112844.htm

163. "Sense of Purpose in Life Linked to Lower Mortality and Cardiovascular Risk," *Wolters Kluwer Health: Lippincott Williams and Wilkins*, Science Daily, last accessed June 2024, https://www.sciencedaily.com/releases/2015/12/151203112844.htm.

164. Dr. Patricia A. Boyle et al, "Effect of Purpose in Life on the Relation Between Alzheimer Disease Pathologic Changes on Cognitive Function in Advanced Age," *Archives of General Psychiatry*, 69 (5), (May 2012): 499–505, https://doi.org/10.1001/archgenpsychiatry.2011.1487.

165. Eric S. Kim et al, "Association Between Purpose in Life and Objective Measures of Physical Function in Older Adults," *JAMA Psychiatry*, 74, (10), (October 2017): 1039–1045, https://doi.org/10.1001/jamapsychiatry.2017.2145.

167. "Live to 100: Secret of the BlueZones,"(2023) Netflix.

168. Robert Wright, "Can Evolution Have a Higher Purpose?" *New York Times*, December 2016, last accessed May 2024, https://www.nytimes.com/2016/12/12/opinion/can-evolution-have-a-higher-purpose.html.

ACKNOWLEDGMENTS

An audacious goal like making aging and illness optional can not be achieved alone. I am deeply thankful for everyone who has made this mission possible and will continue this journey with me. This book has been a key part of our endeavor to share the latest science and inspire others to choose health. If our bodies and minds are healthy, we have a key part of what we need to live a life of purpose where we improve lives, which is the greatest gift anyone can give.

To my dear wife and partner Anu: it is a joy to do this journey with you by my side. Thank you for supporting me, being patient, wise and grounded and supporting another one of my wild ideas.

To my kids, Ankur, Priyanka, and Neil: It has been incredible to watch you grow and launch your own businesses and endeavors to make this world better. I remember when you were kids and would roll your eyes at your dear ol' dad's crazy pursuits. Now you get it. I look forward to continuing to watch you grow and now we can mentor one another as we learn from our various ventures.

Thank you to my incredible team at Viome: We have achieved this together, and we will continue to push the boundaries of precision medicine. To my team—Momo Vuyisich, Guru Banavar, Helene Vollbracht, Stephen Barrie, Sarah Dorsett, and our dedicated clinical team of doctors, scientists, nutritionists, and experts—your contributions have been invaluable in our journey, educating and advancing our research and development. Special thanks to Grant Antoine, Hilary Keiser, and Janelle Connell for being an instrumental part of bringing our personalized formulas to life as we stand at the frontlines of the personalized nutrition revolution.

To our users: When you choose us, you choose yourself and your body. You take ownership, and you are helping shift the paradigm on healthcare to one where the health of each individual is prioritized ahead of profit. I acknowledge you for your commitment to great health. It is not always easy, but it is worth it. Thank you for being part of the movement and contributing to breakthroughs in health sciences.

To my industry peers who care deeply about advancing our knowledge and the field of precision health and longevity: I value how we learn from one another and friendly competitions to grow younger as we get chronologically older. I have learned tremendously from each of you.

To my writing partners who made this book possible: You listened to my stories, dug into the science, and wrapped everything together to create a light, inspiring, and practical read. I am grateful to have you, Kay

Walker, as my book collaborator and Andy Walker as my development editor from the Cyberwalker Media team on this book.

To the publishing team, Igniting Souls: Thank you Kary Obrerunner, Sarah Grandstaff, Ruthie Bult, Jill Ellis, and Elizabeth Haller for your commitment to packaging this book in a way that would translate to our vision and inspire many readers in their health journey. You have been instrumental in positioning us to get the visibility we need to continue to grow our movement towards better health for all.

Let us all stay healthy so we can continue to enjoy many more collaborations and great times together. I thank you deeply for your efforts on this book and as we continue this journey.

ABOUT THE AUTHOR

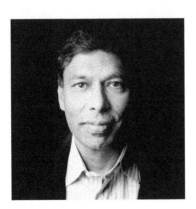

Naveen Jain tackles some of the world's biggest problems with an unshakeable entrepreneurial spirit and a relentless pursuit of seemingly impossible goals.

The term "moonshot" has become synonymous with his name and, by extension, his wildly ambitious projects that include companies in longevity and precision nutrition, Internet search innovations, and lunar logistics and mining.

Driven by his fierce commitment, Jain's company Moon Express became the first company granted permission to land on the Moon, with an even grander objective to conduct lunar mining for rare earth elements and other valuable resources. His current audacious vision is to make aging and illness optional, a goal that is rapidly becoming a reality through his company, Viome Life Sciences. Together with a team of world-class health researchers and scientists, Viome has developed products that empower individuals to take control of their health and nutrition, aiming to help them live longer and free from disease.

Naveen has also founded innovative companies such as the World Innovation Institute, TalentWise, Intelius, and Infospace. His boundless curiosity drives him to embrace bold ideas that propel humanity forward. With an uncanny ability to envision realities beyond what many believe is possible, he pursues unconventional business strategies and harnesses the most advanced technologies to achieve outcomes that leave observers amazed and inspired.

Naveen is the author of the award-winning book *Moonshots: Creating a World of Abundance* and the creator of Mindvalley's *The Power of Boldness* and *Gut Health* masterclasses. He serves as Vice-Chairman of the Board at Singularity University, where his passion lies in educating and inspiring leaders, empowering them to leverage cutting-edge technologies to address humanity's most pressing challenges. As a board member of the XPRIZE Foundation, Naveen actively contributes to pushing the boundaries of possibility through incentivized prize competitions, catalyzing positive change on a global scale.

Naveen's visionary leadership has garnered numerous accolades, reflecting his unwavering dedication and trailblazing spirit. From being recognized as "Entrepreneur of the Year" by Ernst & Young to receiving the esteemed "Most Creative Person" title from Fast Company, his exceptional contributions have left an indelible mark. His brilliance and philanthropic endeavors have earned him prestigious honors, including the esteemed "Lifetime Achievement Award" by Red Herring and the notable "Medal of Honor" by Ellis Island. Notably, Town & Country Magazine celebrated him as one of the "Top 50 Philanthropists," further underscoring his commitment to making a meaningful impact.

In philanthropy, the Naveen & Anu Jain Family Foundation focuses on empowering women and girls, promoting health and wellness, educating youth, and fostering entrepreneurship. Jain is fiercely committed to mentoring the next generation of entrepreneurs to be world-class leaders.

Naveen's mission, whether commercial or philanthropic, is to enhance as many lives as possible. He champions a strategic and systematic approach to philanthropy, applying entrepreneurial principles to create sustainable, impactful change.

CONNECT WITH NAVEEN

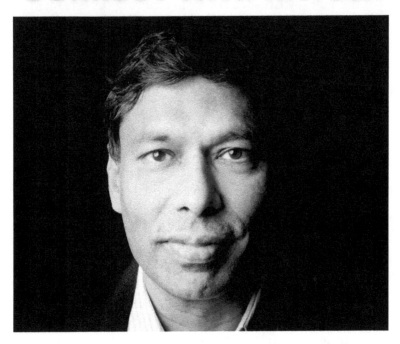

Follow him on your favorite
social media platforms today.

NaveenJain.com

ABOUT VIOME
LIFE SCIENCES

Viome is revolutionizing the field of longevity and preventive healthcare by turning scientific breakthroughs into personalized, practical health solutions. Using cutting-edge AI and the world's largest gene expression database, our at-home- tests provide personalized health insights, nutritional guidance, and personalized microbiome health products to help you live a longer, healthier life. By combining advanced RNA sequencing with AI technology, Viome delivers detailed health insights that guide you throughout your health journey as it evolves towards a vibrant and healthy future.

Our mission is to tackle the root causes of chronic diseases and aging by offering precise nutritional solutions that address the unique needs of each individual, no matter where they are on their health journey.

We've created a true movement in healthcare by bringing together the best minds, science, and technology to simplify the complexities of the human body, making it easier to know just what it needs. Our mission is to empower our users to take control of their health using data-driven insights rather than guesswork. We believe in clear, transparent communication that educates and empowers, transforming health from a confusing puzzle into a manageable journey. Imagine a future where medicine comes from farms, not pharmacies, and healthcare happens at home, not in hospitals.

At Viome, we believe that insights are only valuable when they lead to actionable steps you can use daily to make little changes that have big long-term benefits. Our innovative approach includes using state-of-the-art robotics to create custom-formulated supplements tailored to your unique needs. By addressing the nutritional gaps identified in your Viome test results, our evidence-based formulas provide the exact dosages and ingredients your microbiome requires.

We are committed to using data for the good of humanity, continuously giving back to our users by transforming what we learn into new lifesaving tests, better insights, more advanced personalization capabilities, and new innovative products. From early detection of microbial signals that precede symptoms to early detection of life-threatening diseases and cancers, Viome is dedicated to uncovering the root causes of health challenges and paving the way for new preventative strategies. Join us in redefining health and wellness for a future where you have the power to thrive. For more information, visit: Viome.com.

Imagine a World Where Aging is Optional

Learn More

TheYouthFormula.com

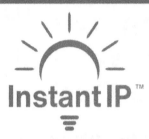